The Pelvic Book for Osteopaths and Chiropractors

Good science begins from a starting point that is pure and uncontaminated from other people's misconceptions and prejudices. Bad science sets out from a mid-point and builds on the misconceptions and prejudices that have gone before.

The science behind this book starts from the very beginning and provides a step by step set of new theories on how the pelvis articulates in a way that conforms with true human joint movements. It then covers the forces that create sacroiliac and iliosacral lesions and how they go on to create the 'pelvic lesion' that locks them in. Lastly, a procedure for correcting the pelvic lesion.

No research or theory has ever come this close to understanding the physiology of the pelvic joints, let alone identified the underlying pelvic lesion in such detail.

A

The Pelvic Book for Osteopaths and Chiropractors

Other publications by J.R.Bayliss:

DVD: Spinal Mechanics and Bony Locking *For Health Professionals*
by John Bayliss DO and Peter O'Toole
ISBN 0-9550936-0-0

Book: The Theory of Synergetic Spinal Mechanics and PPT Manipulation
by John Bayliss
Out of print

Book: The Theory of Synergetic Spinal Mechanics and PPT Manipulation
Edition 2

by J.R. Bayliss
ISBN 0-9550936-2-7

Book: Advanced Osteopathic Technique
(PPT Manipulation and synergetic bio-mechanics)

by J.R. Bayliss
ISBN 978-0-9550936-3-5

Published by: John Bayliss
3, Moor Lane
Chessington
Surrey KT9 1BJ
England UK
www.spinalmechanics.com

ISBN 978-0-9550936-7-8

Background to this book by J.R.Bayliss.

"In 2005, I worked out how the pelvis and spine interact in harmony to produce real world, human movement. I was also able to explain for the first time in Osteopathic/ Chiropractic history, how the S/I and spinal joints become so locked against each other that they force bone against bone, which is the essence of an Osteopathic lesion. (Chiropractic subluxation).

Since then, knowing how facet joints lock against each other, it was possible for me to work out a method of manipulation that reversed the forces that create an Osteopathic lesion. I called the new ground-breaking techniques PPT's (passive patient technique). With PPT's there are no contorted patient positions, no clicks, and have high accuracy. They work every time. They are fast, simple to apply and genuinely long lasting. My books, the last one was titled 'Advanced Osteopathic Technique' have sold all over the world.

However, there was one area that I felt needed to be covered in more detail, and that was the '**Pelvic Lesion**'. It is the physical manipulative professions most poorly recognized and understood lesion. It was thought that by correcting the sacroiliac and iliosacral lesions with classical manipulative techniques, the correct mobility and alignment of the pelvis would yield the best possible results. However, the underlying 'pelvic lesion', which reinforces and locks-in the sacroiliac lesions on weight bearing, was overlooked. This meant that on weight bearing all the corrected S/I and I/O lesions reappear".

Acknowledgments

I would like to thank all the people who encouraged me to write this book, in particular Juraj Prvy who gave me the motivation, and John Day for his professional contribution on page 21.

Behind the camera: Daniel Bayliss
                                  Peter O' Tool.

Front Cover design: Daniel Bayliss

Editing and technical consultant .   Juraj Prvy

_____

About the Author J.R.Bayliss
J.R.Bayliss DO is a retired UK Osteopath who trained with the 'College of Osteopaths Educational Trust.' He has a background in engineering and worked out all the real world mechanics behind the way the pelvis articulates and lesions from an engineering point of view. He envisaged and drew all of the illustrations.

C

Introduction

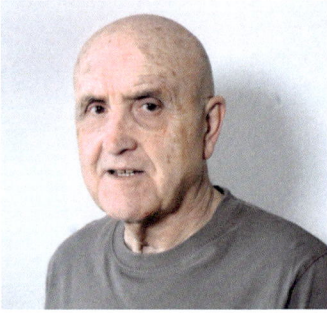

John R Bayliss

"When I studied Osteopathy back in the eighties no one could tell us in bony terms what an Osteopathic lesion was in any meaningful way. That was still the case until I wrote my modern comprehensive book 'Advanced Osteopathic Technique' (AOT). Before, we had been given fancy quotes from famous Osteopaths about the soft tissue changes they thought took place, but nothing about how the joints themselves physically locked against each other.

For example, we were taught that a spinal lesion can be side-bent left and rotated right, or rotated and side-bent right etc...but that was how H. Fryette who was in vogue at the time described spinal articulation. (His work has since been disproved by imaging results). Something was clearly missing, and until my work had never been meaningfully addressed.

The old thinking on the mechanics of the sacroiliac joints was based on imaged research that was clearly carried out on lesioned joint facets. The simple semi-dislocation articulation the research concluded is still held as sterling by some, because it was 'researched' and the underlying 'pelvic lesion' was never mentioned. This unawareness remained at the time of writing this book. There was clearly a vacuum of knowledge within the professions that was being glossed over.

Building on the information I had accumulated from writing my book (AOT), with the aid of a dissected pelvis, I set out to discover for myself how 'pelvic lesions' occur from a mechanical engineering point of view. How they self-perpetuate, and how to correct. To my knowledge no one has ever come close to doing this before and it gives me great pleasure after many years to finally be able to share something I am so passionate about."

This book takes the reader through each and every step, so the reader can see for themselves why my theories are valid. A myriad of photographs and illustrations accompany the detailed explanations.

Correcting the pelvic lesion is the most profound treatment an Osteopath or Chiropractor can give their patient, as the changes made to the musculo-skeletal frame are significant. As it has never been fully understood, before, those who learn to correct the 'Pelvic lesion' will be amongst an elite minority.

"John's previous book on spinal mechanics (AOT) made a big change to my thinking and how I practiced. Before I would research an area, but then I found none of the research linked to other areas. Learning John's work helped me to understand the complete picture, where all the joints synchronized. I travelled to England to meet John for a workshop and we have since becomes friends. My patients as a result of my new knowledge are getting better and straighter much quicker, and for longer. With so much misinformation available online and in outdated books, I was proud to offer my assistance in the making of this truly pioneering book."

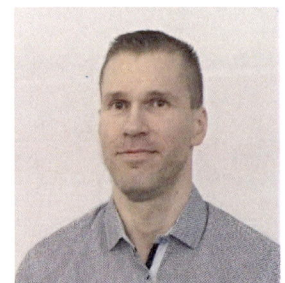

Juraj Prvy

Index

E

Index

Chapter One
Introduction into how the pelvis was designed to work

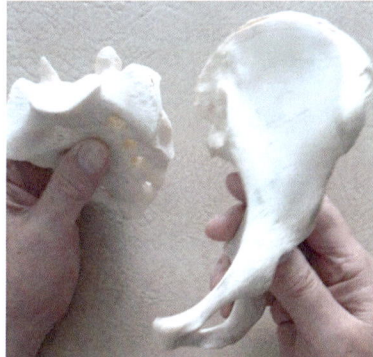

Figure P1

The Pelvis

Pelvic lesions are very common but poorly understood, and rarely corrected. Correcting a sacroiliac and Iliosacral lesion does not correct the underlying pelvic lesion. A pelvic lesion locks in the sacroiliac and iliosacral lesions. If the pelvic lesion is not corrected, the sacroiliac and iliosacral lesions that have just been corrected will return to their former lesioned position on weight bearing.

This chapter introduces you to the design and physiology of the sacroiliac joints from an engineering point of view. If you want to know how the pelvis relates to the rest of the body, this very important information is detailed in my book '**Advanced Osteopathic technique**'.

The pelvis is a very important component of the human body and plays a vital role in the function and articulation of the whole spine, as well as directing leg movements. Due to a lack of experimentation from an engineering point of view by the physical professions, how the pelvis articulated has remained a mystery to all of them.

Before any valid research can take place, there has to be a working model, which until my books, was not available to Osteopaths or Chiropractors.

The pelvis and spine work together in a flowing harmonious action. If you take one or two items which I was told valid research requires, it would be like taking one or two gears out of a car gearbox and trying to make sense of how the gear box works in harmony with all the other mechanisms that work together to drive the car, and how the car malfunctions.

Published research has focused in on the internal articulation of the sacroiliac joints without reference to their function. Many authorities have accepted this research in good faith without thinking it through for themselves, because it was "researched" using highly accurate imaging techniques. The problem is this published research describes the facets in a state of semi-dislocation with no reference to the mayhem that causes. **Sacroiliac joints are not designed to semi-dislocate** with every step a human takes.

On a positive note, the results from sacroiliac imaging focus research has brought to the surface what the medical profession question and deny even exist. An Osteopathic sacroiliac lesion/ chiropractic subluxation.

Overview

Important overview

There are many misconceptions about the way the pelvis articulates. This book looks at the pelvic articulations purely from an engineering point of view to give the reader a fundamental understanding of how the pelvis accomplishes the many tasks it is set.

Misconceptions:

1 What is referred to as 'nutation' is not a front to back arc of the iliac crest moving anterio-inferiorly and then posterio-superiorly. The apparent "nutation" affect is mimicked by the angle of the iliac facets and iliac crest oscillating like a fan medially and then laterally in opposite directions.

2 The sacrum does not have a memory inside it that magically slides the sacral facets into the correct position. The sacroiliac joint is not designed to be a sliding joint. It is an oblong contact joint. There are <u>no</u> muscles locally or distally that would cause any kind of structured minute sacroiliac articulations.

Things you need to know:

3 The sacrum acts as a see-saw pinion between the two Ilia. It is powered by the side-shift movements of the pelvis.

4 The point of contact made along the sacroiliac facets via pelvic side-shift, determines the position of the acetabulum and legs.

5 The Iliac facets have a middle division running along its length that divides the facets into a superior half and an inferior half. The superior half of the iliac facets are designed for weight bearing, and the lower facets to act as a guide for the leading leg to go forward.

6 The symphysis pubis stabilises the inferior part of pelvis and acts as a push-pull lever joint.

7 Some will say, where is your research and imagine they are being impressive? And I would say to that *I see you have a nose on the front of your face, because it is self-eviden*t. The way joints articulate is self-evident providing you know what drives them and their function. Basic common sense and applied physics need to come before research. History has proved that.

How the pelvis articulates is based on many elements working altogether in harmony with each other. *Not in isolation, as research favours*. Each element is vitally important in its own right. Professionals need to have an overall understanding of how the pelvis, legs, and spine articulate in harmony, and synergetically with each other before they can begin their research. This is what my advanced work pioneered back 2005. I made a film, so it could be seen with your very own eyes. I showed for the very first time in the history of Osteopathy and Chiropractic, what an Osteopathic lesion was on a bony level (facet against facet), and how they become locked-in. The very science the professions so badly need to know.

Anatomy of the ilium

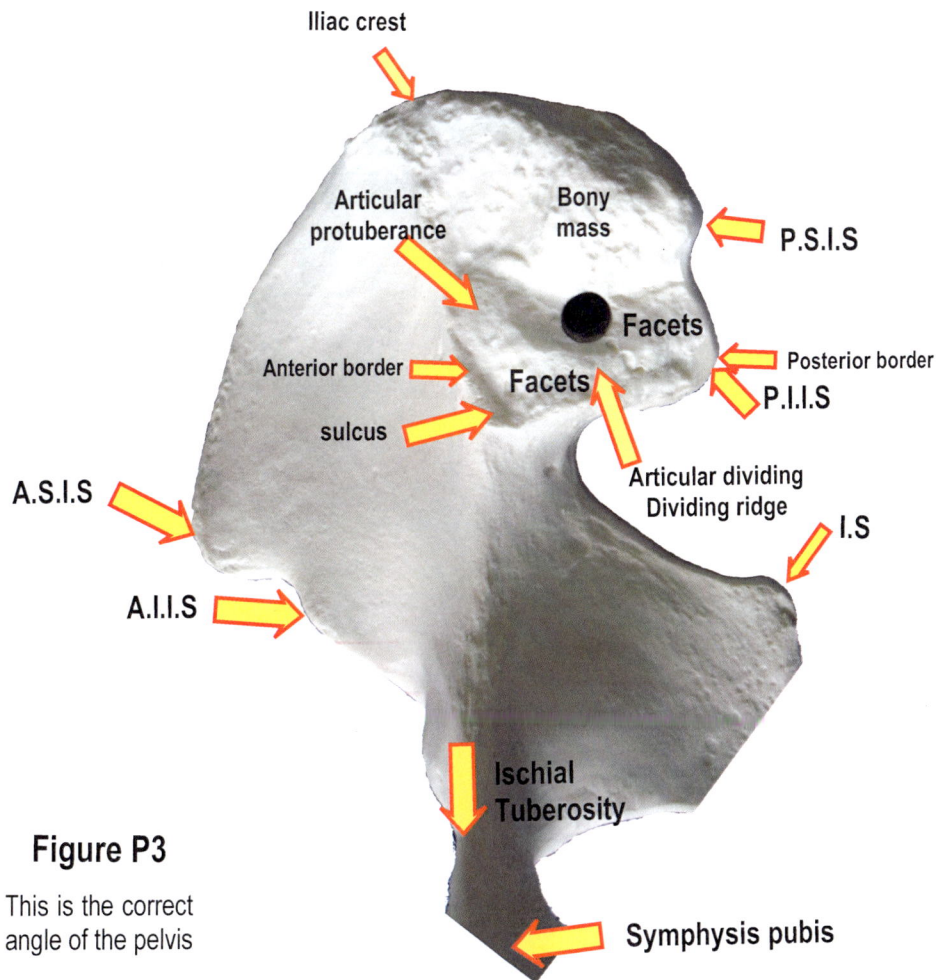

Iliac crest

Articular protuberance

Bony mass

P.S.I.S

Facets

Anterior border

Facets

Posterior border

P.I.I.S

sulcus

A.S.I.S

Articular dividing
Dividing ridge

I.S

A.I.I.S

Ischial
Tuberosity

Figure P3

This is the correct
angle of the pelvis

Symphysis pubis

Figure P3 Innominate land marks

The sacroiliac joint

There are many variations in the shapes and sizes of the sacroiliac articular facets. However, all sacroiliac facet shapes share certain common similarities and these are explained further in this chapter. **Figure P3** shows a plastic mould of a right Ilium and details the main names of the bony architecture.

At the superior border of the Iliac facet there is a bony mass that would if dislocation took place buffer excessive weight bearing. Dividing the Iliac facets in half is a horizontal bony ridge that runs along the middle. In the example above, there is a deep sulcus at the anterio-inferior border to prohibit excessive inferior sacral movement. In other types of facets, the anterior ridge of the sulcus is less pronounced or missing. A more pronounced dividing ridge will produce a more efficient walking and running gait, whereas a flatter ridge would produce a type of mincing gait more suited to swimming and cycling.

The angle of the pelvis is approximately as you see it here. At this angle the facets line up along the gravity line of the acetabulum below. This gravity line changes constantly during weight bearing and walking.

The iliac facet names

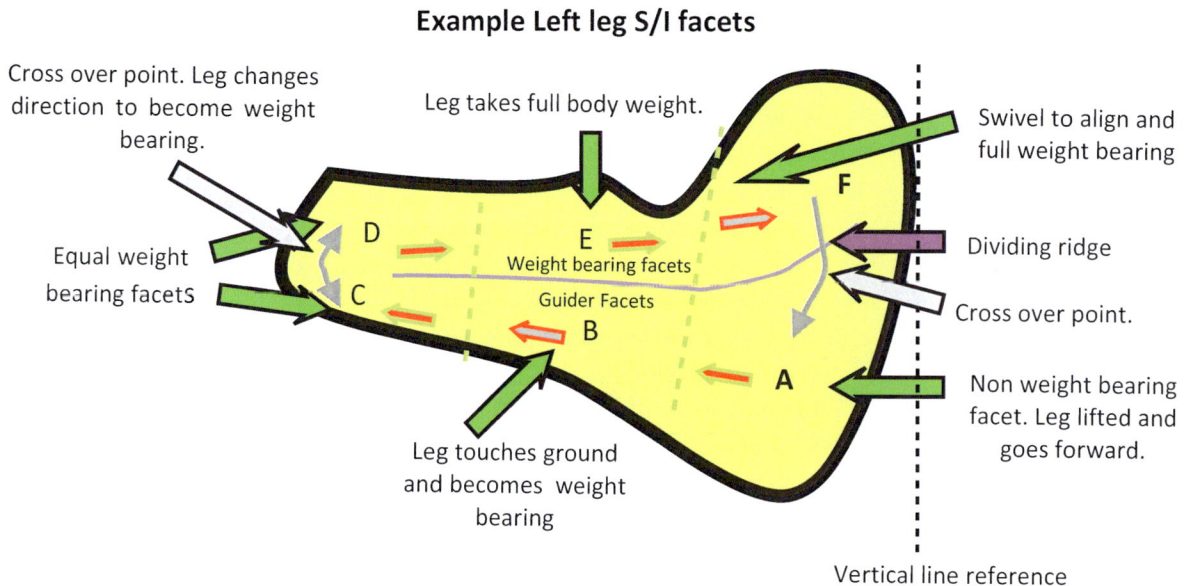

Example Left leg S/I facets

Cross over point. Leg changes direction to become weight bearing.

Leg takes full body weight.

Swivel to align and full weight bearing

F

Equal weight bearing facetS

D

E
Weight bearing facets

Guider Facets

C

B

A

Dividing ridge

Cross over point.

Non weight bearing facet. Leg lifted and goes forward.

Leg touches ground and becomes weight bearing

Vertical line reference

Figure P4 is an illustration of an Iliac facet. The red arrows show the path the leading leg takes to become weight bearing.

The Iliac facet

The iliac facets are horizontally divided down the middle by a mildly raised dividing ridge. This ridge allows for two way traffic above and below. One leg stays put while the other goes forward. Two opposite directions.

It is important to note that the sacroiliac joint is not a sliding joint. It is an elongated contact joint.

Whilst the facet in **figure P4** is shown in six segments for simplicity, the whole surface is in contact. Movement is caused by pelvic side-shift and the reactive ground forces acting on each segment.

According to the Bayliss synergetic theory, the 'A' to 'C' facets are guider facets, and the 'D' to 'F' facets are the weight bearing facets.

Figure P4. During walking with the left leg leading, follow the red arrows:

1 The left leg is angled and raised and goes forward as the left S/I 'A' facet is engaged.

2 The left leg touches the ground and takes mild weight bearing at the 'B' facet.

3 When the left leg is at the midpoint, the 'C' facet is engaged, see **figure P8**. (Up to now the left leg has been moving forward).

4 As the leg becomes more weight bearing having passed over the 'D' facet, the full body weight is taken on the 'E' facet.

5 The full body weight is swivelled from the 'E' facet to the 'F' facet to align the pelvis.

On the right leg, the S/I facets travel in the opposite direction. See green arrows. Refer to **figure P8 and P7D**.

How the facets are powered

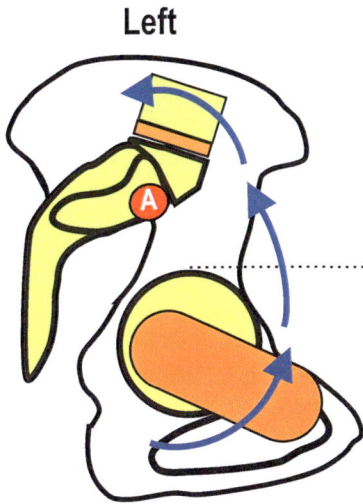

Left   **Right**

Figure P5A Illustration

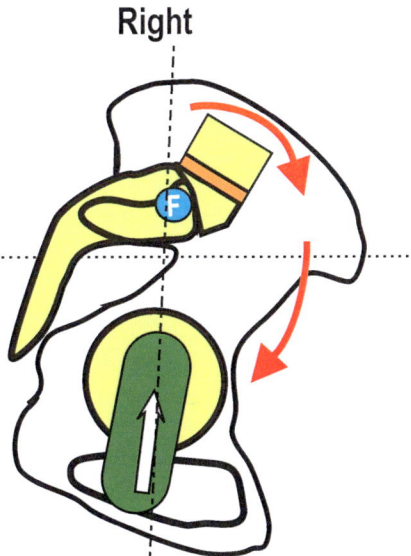

Figure P5B Illustration

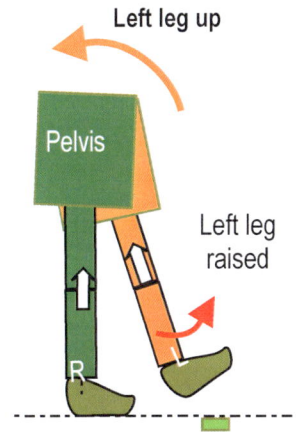

Left leg up

Pelvis

Left leg raised

R

Figure P5 A+B Illustration

Sacrum acts as horizontal lever

Sacroiliac joint facet articulation is powered by side-shift and weight distribution, not muscle. See **page 17**. The sacrum acts as a guiding lever between the iliac facets.

Figure P5AA is a diagram of the sacrum in neutral.

Figure P5BB is a diagram of the sacrum as pelvic side-shift transfers to the right. The reactive force travels up the right leg to engage the right Iliac 'F' facet on the sacral 'F' facet. This puts a body weight transfer of force across the sacrum to engage the non-weight bearing left 'A' sacroiliac facets. This lifts the left ilium.

Illustrations P5A, P5B, and P5A+B show how the engagement of the facets translate into leg placement.

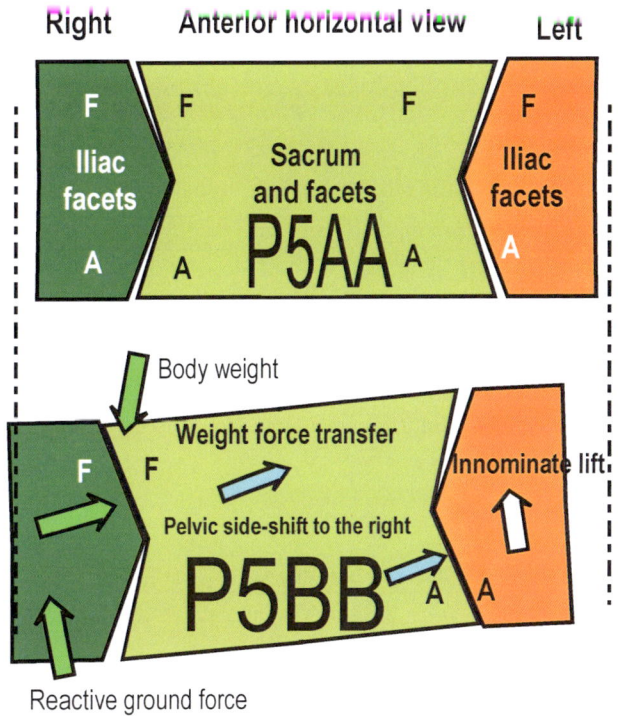

Right   Anterior horizontal view   **Left**

F   F   F   F

Iliac facets   Sacrum and facets   Iliac facets

A   A   P5AA   A   A

Body weight

Weight force transfer

F   F   Innominate lift

Pelvic side-shift to the right

P5BB   A   A

Reactive ground force

Figures P5 AA-BB illustrate how the sacrum communicates and guides the iliac facets on either side.

5

Breakdown of iliac facet surfaces

The four illustrations below show the exaggerated main components of iliac facet surfaces.

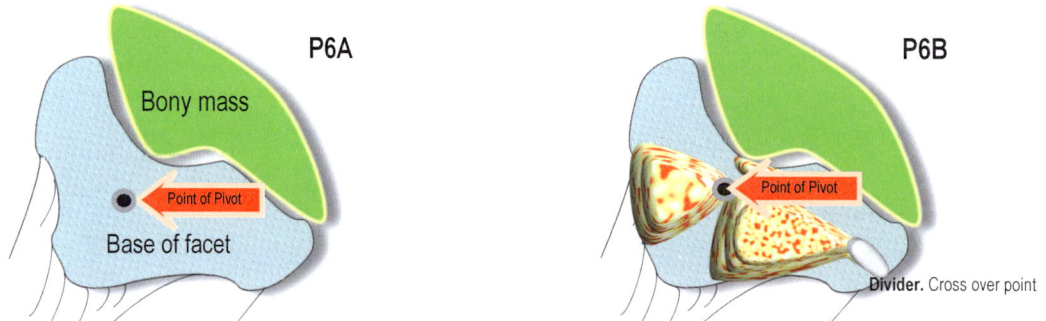

Figure P6A provides a closer look at an Iliac facet without any contours or articular surfaces added. The bony mass shown in green acts as a buffer should too much weight be placed on facets 'D-F'.

In **figure P6B** the irregular spotted yellow area shown is the divider ridge that runs along the middle of the facet. At first sight the contours look like a design by committee. However, these contours are designed to play an important placement role. The point of pivot is the area engaged when the sacrum is in neutral.

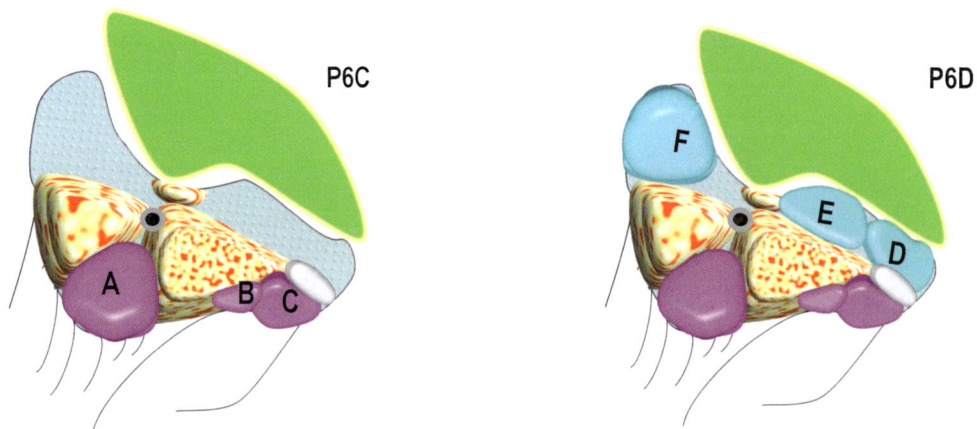

In **figure P6C** the inferior guider facets, shown in purple are designed to angle and align the leading leg during walking etc. They form a complex elongated contact joint. *Facet A* is the true anterior articular surface and is there to guide the thigh/leg forward, medially and upward in a non-weight-bearing capacity. *Facet B* has a transitory function and is there to guide the thigh/leg towards the ground. Once the foot touches the ground, *facet* C acts as a transitory weight bearing cross-over point to the transitory load bearing *facet D,* shown in **figure P6D.** At this point the weight of the body is taken equally on both feet.

Figure P6D. As more weight is transferred to the supporting leg, the reactive upward ground-resistance causes the transitory weight bearing *facet E* to engage. Finally, when the full weight of the body is taken on the supporting vertical leg, the meeting of the ground-resistance returning up the leg causes the main load bearing *facet F* to engage. Note the angle of the 'F' facet is opposite the 'A' facet. The whole surface of the S/I joint facets are articulator surfaces. The highlighted six are the main ones.

The iliac facet angles

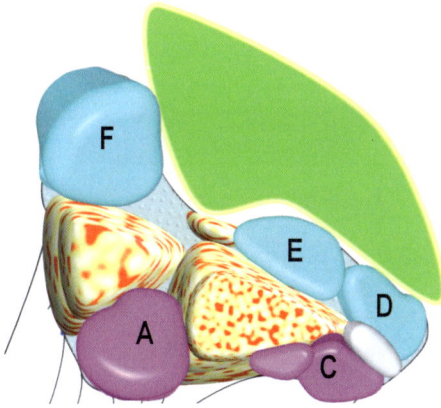

Figure 7A is an illustration of the angles
of the F and A facets

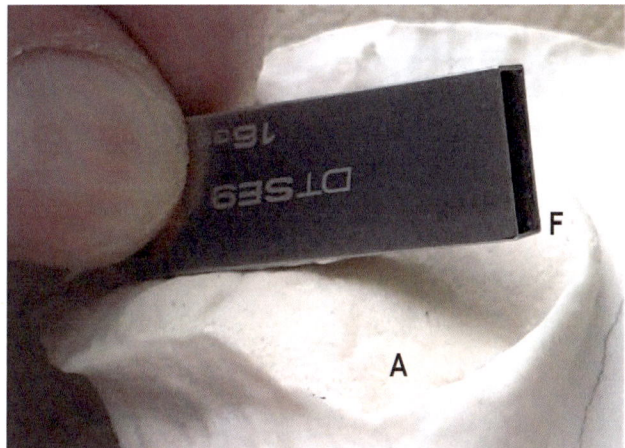

Figure 7B is a side view of the angles of the F and A
facets on a sacrum.

The 'F' facet design

The 'F' and 'A' facets are designed for two different
purposes.   The 'F' facet is angled inferiorly to push
the ilium laterally and inferiorly. The 'A' facet is
designed to align and lift the ilium.

Figure 7A, is a simple illustration of the angles of
the 'F' and 'A' facets. Note the height of the ridge
between the 'F' and 'A' facet can vary in some
people from a minor bump to a pronounced ridge.

Figure 7B, is a side-posterior view of the 'F' and 'A'
facets on a young persons real sacrum. This is to
further illustrate the different angles of the 'F' and
'A' facets.

Figure 7C, is a side-horizontal view of the 'F' and 'A'
facets on a real ilium. Note the rounded steep
incline from facets 'E' to 'F' and 'A' to 'B'. This is to
accommodate the swivel action illustrated in **figure
P10B**.

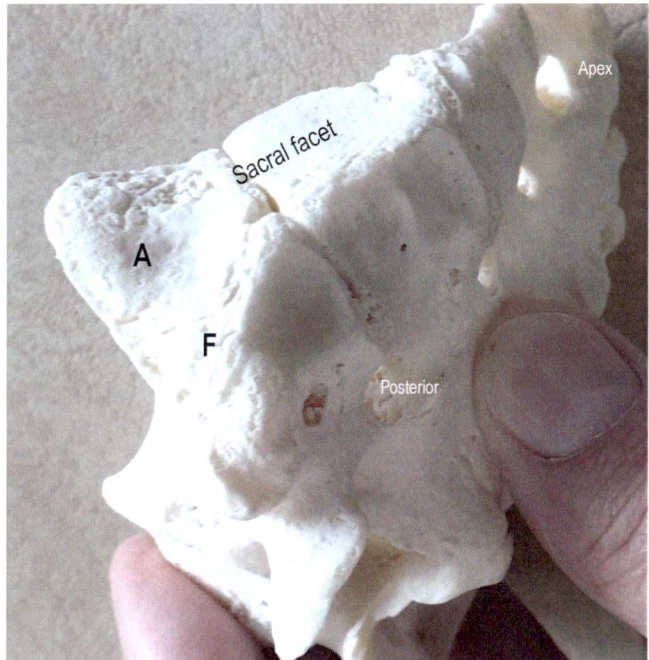

Figure 7C is a horizontal view of the angles of the iliac
E to F facets.

An introduction into the design of the sacroiliac facets - Part one

Mechanics behind the design of the sacroiliac joints

The sacroiliac facets do not physically slide up and down or slide around on each other. They have multi-faceted surfaces that come into contact through pelvic side-shift and weight distribution.

Walking test. Stand up on your right leg with the intention of walking. To do this and keep your balance, you had to side-shift your pelvis to the right. As you did this, your pelvis swivelled to the right and lifted the left side of your pelvis, which in turn, lifted, swivelled, and angled your left leg/foot to align straight ahead.

With muscle help, move your left leg forward as you would in your normal walking stride. As you put your left foot to the ground your weight distribution changes. As your left foot becomes weight bearing, your pelvis will be in your body's mid-line. Equal body weight is now taken on both feet. Left facet 'C' and right facet 'D'.

As your body weight transfers to the left leg and you precede forward, your pelvis arcs to the left and swivels at the "F" facet.

The two pelvic arcs

The pelvic movement you have just confirmed is shown in **figure P8** (Feet are shown in blue and pelvis in faded red and green). You can see two distinct tracking radii on either side. The 'X' and 'Y' arcs. Arc 'Y' has a tighter radius than arc 'X'. This tells us that the sacroiliac facets would need two different articulatory contoured surfaces in order to account for this difference. Notice that there

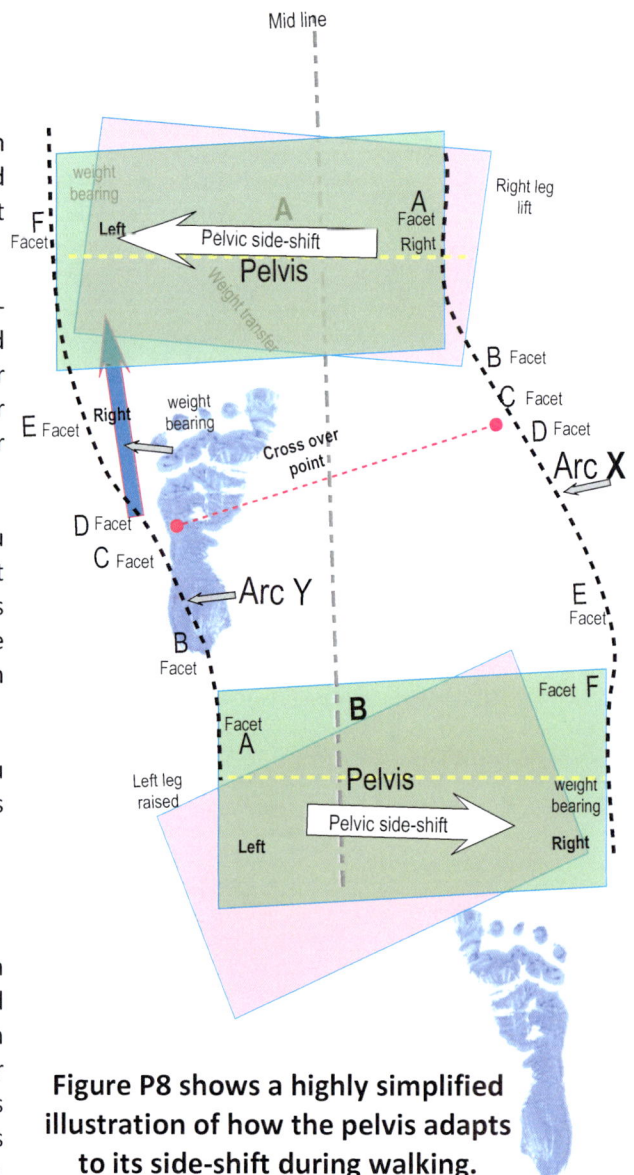

Figure P8 shows a highly simplified illustration of how the pelvis adapts to its side-shift during walking.

are three crossover points shown in **figure P8.** These points illustrate where weight and side-shift cross over from each other. One point is within each pelvis (shown by yellow dotted arrows) and one midway between(shown as a red dotted arrow). If we remove one pelvis to simplify, there are two crossover points:

1) One within the pelvis. (Full weight bearing with side-shift on one side taken on facet F. See page 6).

2) One midway between a leg stride. (Equal weight distribution facets C/D. See **figure P16C**).

The sacroiliac facets have to account for factors 1) and 2). It is logical to assume that the cross over point where the full body weight is taken on one leg that the facet would be large and sturdy. Whereas at the mid cross over point where body weight is equally distributed on both legs, the facets would be smaller.

An introduction into the design of the sacroiliac facet - Part two

Sacral facet design

If we were to design a facet shape to accommodate the walking action, we would expect the facets from the mid-way point where both legs take equal weight in the midline to become larger as full body weight takes place on one leg. We can speculate that the facets would be pear shaped, see **figure P9A**.

For completeness we will do another self-test to prove the existence of the mid-way facet crossover point.

The guider facet 'A' See page 6, also has a large surface area. To lift the innominate and direct the 'B' facet to guide the leading leg.

The pear shape

The pear shape shown in **figure P9A** vaguely resembles a typical S/I facet and confirms the design of a weight bearing end and a medium weight bearing end.

Next, we need to look at how the S/I joints account for the differences in the radial arcs.

Figure P9B is a photograph of the left sacral facet surfaces. Two radial arcs can be found running parallel along the facet surfaces. One is convex and the other concave. We need to look at why this is. Compare with **figure P8**.

Figure P9C illustrates the sacral facet's crossover points. Weight bearing 'F' rocks over to the 'A' facet. 'C' facet rocks over to the "D" facet.

Not all S/I facets are shaped exactly the same. Some have more or less convexity than others and some have more or less concavity or a mixture of both. Every human has an individual gait.

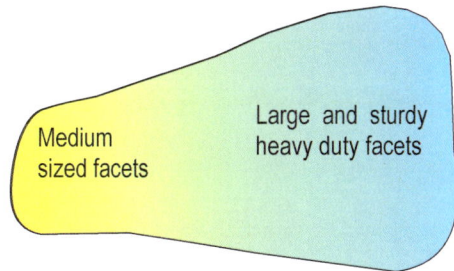

Figure P9A Illustrates the theoretical shape of a sacral facet and the logical areas where cross might take place

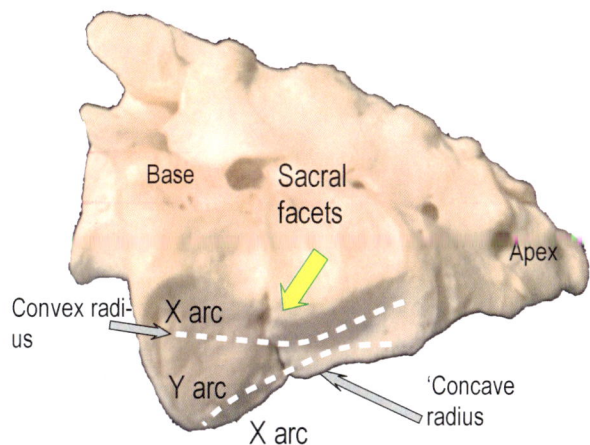

Figure P9B is a a side-view photograph of the left sacral facet surfaces to illustrate the existence of the convex 'Y' radius the concave 'X' radius

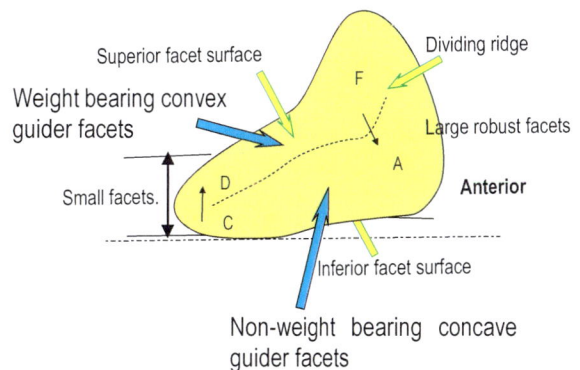

Figure P9C Side-view of a sacral facet

9

The alignment of the feet

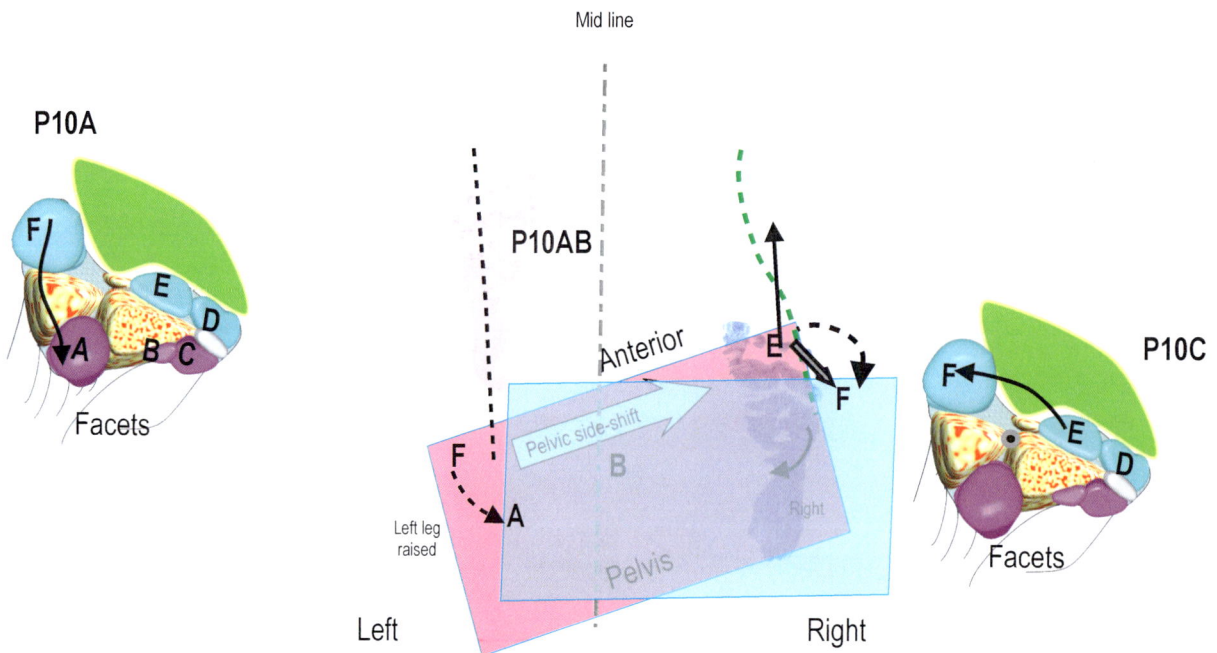

Figure P10B shows the side-shift swivelling action that takes place at the pelvis when body weight side shifts from the right 'E' facet to the right 'F' facet. In order to align the left acetabulum, legs and feet.

Mechanics behind the design of the sacroiliac joints to keep the legs and feet in a straight line.

The feet once they touch the ground do not move. Therefore, all accommodation has to take place via the pelvis during walking.

Do this self-test before proceeding: Stand and transfer your body weight onto your right leg while flexing your non weight bearing left knee. Your pelvis naturally moves laterally and swivels to the right. As shown in **figure P10B**.

In summary:

See **figure 10B**. As the pelvis side-shifts to the right it pushes the right ilium to the right.

This causes the right 'E' facets contact to change to the 'F' facets, see **figure P10C**. This in turn causes the right ASIS to angle laterosuperiorly as the ilium swivels to the right. To align the left side.

The left ilium is dragged medially and is angled to the right.

With the right 'F' facets engaged ecliptically, the left 'A' facets engage. This combined action aligns the left acetabulum and legs/feet on the correct trajectory for the person to walk straight.

This action depends on the sacroiliac joints being in their correct position. If the angles are displaced as in an Osteopathic lesion, the gait will go off alignment.

Innominate angle

Incorrect	Correct	Change in Symphysis pubis

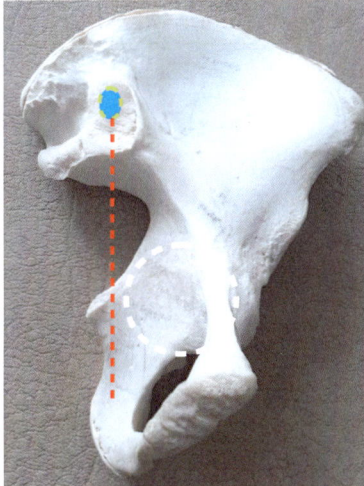

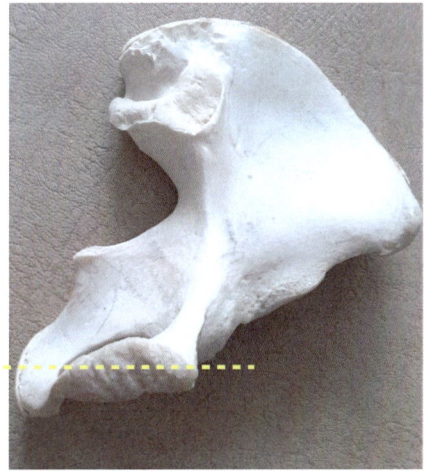

Figure P11A. Photo showing incorrect angle of innominate. Gravity line does not pass through the acetabulum.

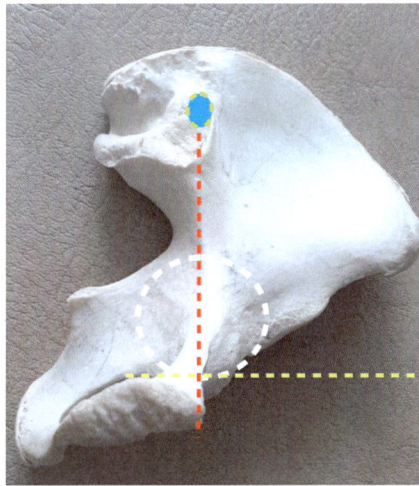

Figure P11B. Photo showing the correct angle of the pelvis. This angle allows the 'F' facet gravity line to pass through the posterior part of the acetabulum.

Figure P11C. Photo showing the change in the angle of the symphysis pubis when weight is placed on the left leg and the pelvis swivels. See next page. Figure P12B.

Working angle of the pelvis

Figure P11A. In anatomy books you will see many photos of the Innominate in this unnatural upright position. In this position the 'F' facet shown in blue would pass a gravity line, shown in red. This line would pass directly downwards and miss the acetabulum altogether and buckle the pelvis.

It's a pretty obvious point yet missed by so many.

Figure P11B. In this figure, from the 'F' facet we see that the angle would look something like this.

Figure P11C, is a photo to show the change in the angle of left the pubic bone after the reactive force has travelled up the leg and swivelled to arrive at the S/I 'F' facet. As shown in **figure P12B** on the following page. (Though it is shown on the right).

Pelvic side-shift and swivel

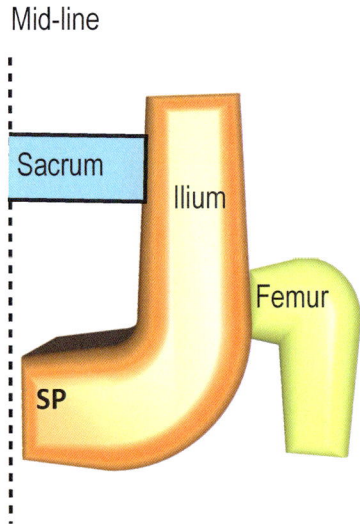

Figure P12A. Posterior view of right pelvis in Neutral.

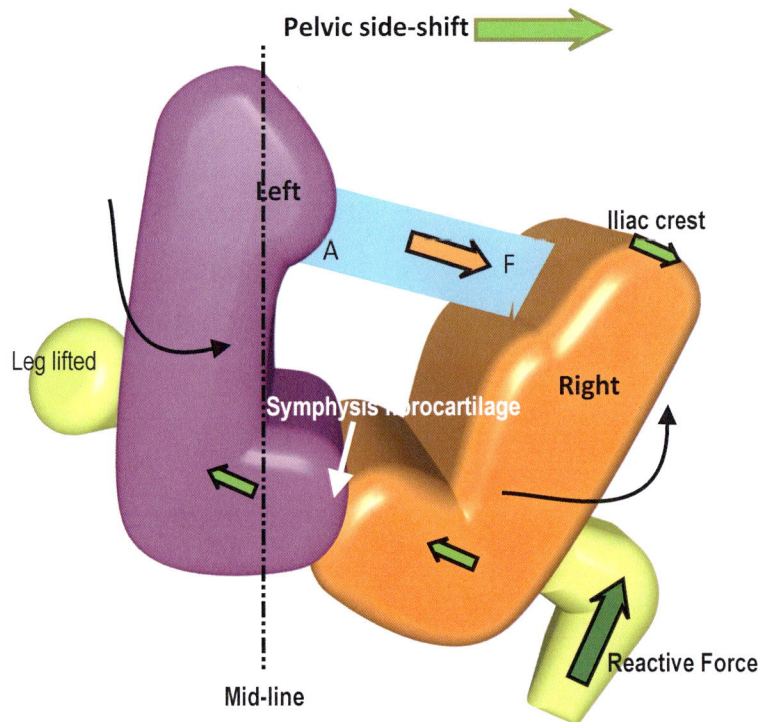

Figure P12B, is a posterior illustration of the pelvis when rotation takes place when weight bearing is taken on the right leg with pelvic side-shift to the right.

Pelvic rotation left when pelvic side-shift is to the right and swivel of the right facets travel: 'E' to 'F'. This is how it was designed to work.

Figure P12A is an illustration for reference only.

Figure 12B, is a crude illustration that shows the changes that occur in the innominates when the pelvis side-shifts to the right and away from the midline and the reactive ground force returns up the right femur. With the right foot fixed and weight bearing, the femoral head is forced laterally at a lateral angle to accommodate the side-shift. This action is caused by the right S/I joint facets as they change from 'E' to 'F' to swivel the right pubic bone towards the left and superior at the symphysis pubis.

The pubic bone on the left is pulled closer to the midline as the S/I 'A' facets are engaged.

The reactive force travelling up the right femur lifts the left innominate and femur off the ground via the 'A' facet and symphysis pubis.

Observation of an innominate

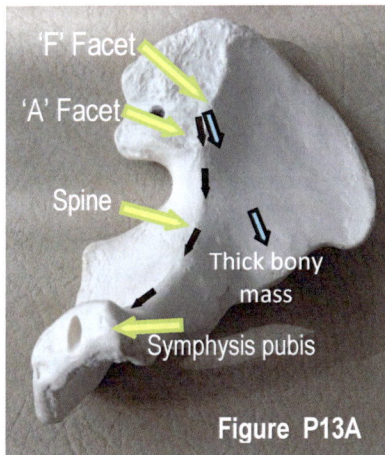

Figure P13A

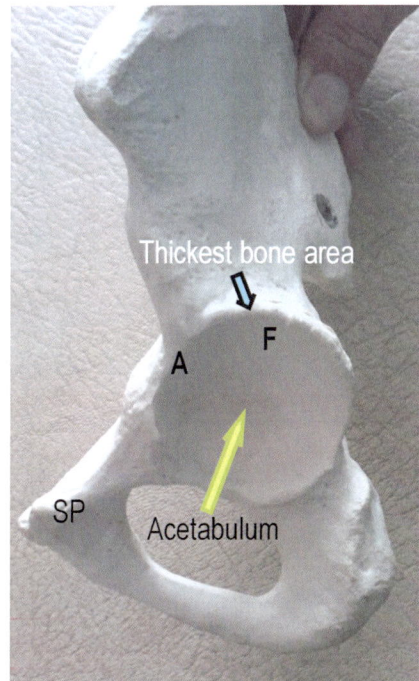

Figure P13B illustrates the approx. areas corresponding to the S/I facets

Points of stress

Figure P13A, is a photo of the inner surface of a typical innominate. Observe the spine shown with black arrows reinforcing the innominate. It runs from below the 'F' and 'A' facets to the symphysis pubis. This spine shows where the stress would be taken during side-shift. The symphysis pubis binds the two innominates together in a stabilizing cushioning way.

The blue arrows shown in **figure P13A** show the linking route from the S/I facets to the acetabulum where the femoral head makes contact.

Figure P13B, shows the approximate area at the perimeter of the acetabulum that correspond to the S/I facets.

Figure P13C, illustrates the vertical wedge shape of the sacrum to block vertical body weight. It narrows medially towards the inferior surface.

Figure P13D, illustrates the horizontal wedge shape of the sacrum to block horizontal body weight slipping between the innominates.

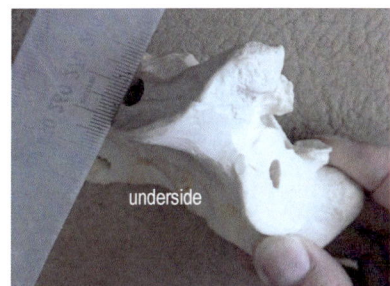

Figure P13C illustrates the angle of the sacral facets

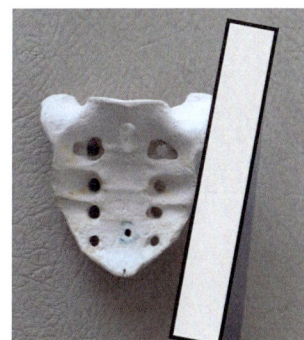

Figure P13D illustrates the horizontal off set angle of the sacral facets

Innominate positions as the facets move to accommodate pelvic side-shift and forward motion.

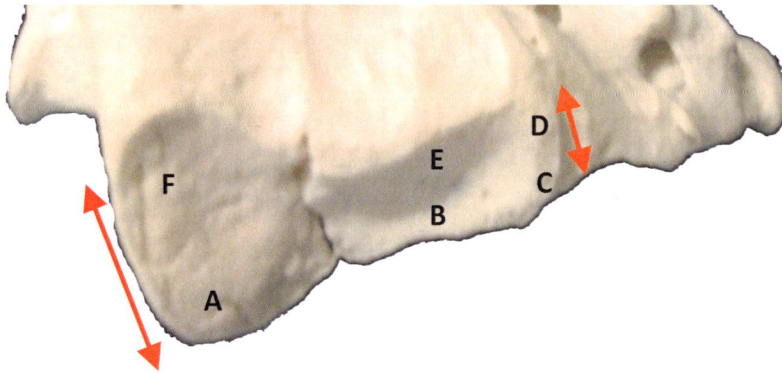

Figure P14A is a side view of a sacrum with the facet reference points added. See how the contours match the walking stride.

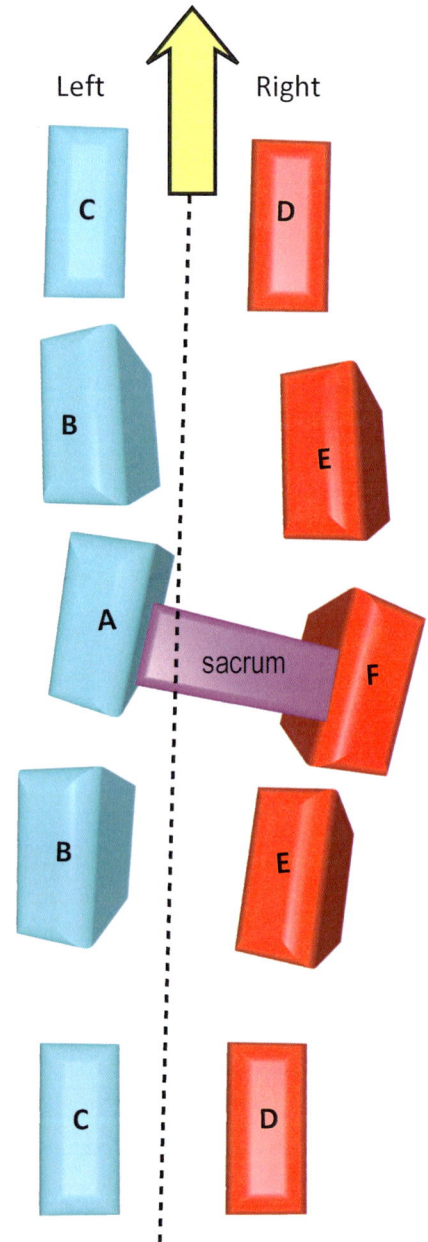

Figure P14A and **B** illustrate the positions of the innominates from above and how the angles of the sacral facets direct the human walking stride when combined with weight bearing and pelvic side-shift.

Before reading this refer t**o figures P4, P7C, P8,** and **P13C.**

Figure P14A. Is a side-view of a typical sacrum. The facet area names have been added.

Figure P14B Is an illustration from above of the angles of left and right side innominates during the walking stride. The distance between the 'F' and 'A' facets is the widest as seen in **figures P14A** and **P7B** at their crossover point.

The facets are at their closest at the 'C' to 'D' crossover point. This is where both legs take equal body weight in the walking stride. **See figure P8**.

Figure P14A and **B** are the positions of the innominates not the feet.

Figure P14B illustrating is an exaggerated view from above of the innominate's during the walking stride.

Bony mass triangle

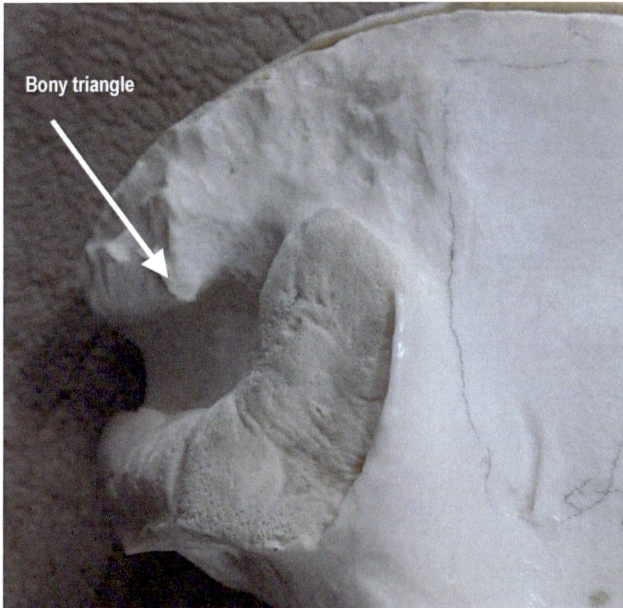

Figure P15A shows the bony triangle that hangs down above the "E-B" facets.

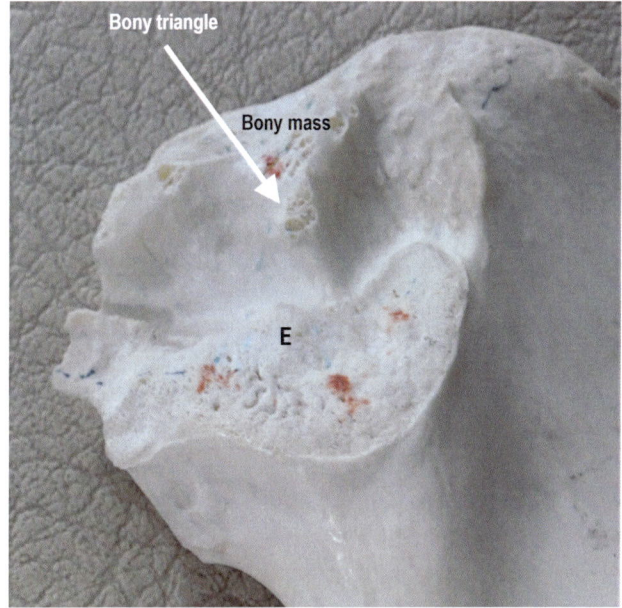

Figure P15B shows the bony triangle that hangs down at around the "E-B" facets on a different ilium.

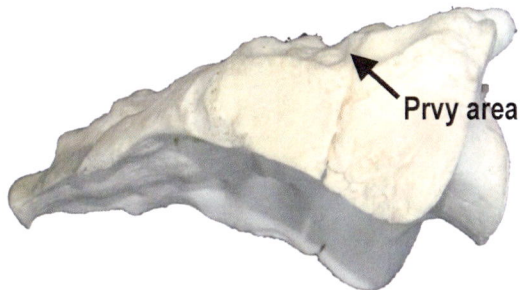

Figure P15C shows the side of a sacral facet to illustrate the extra sacral bony width above the facets. This area is named the 'Prvy' and shown in red on pages 32 and 50.

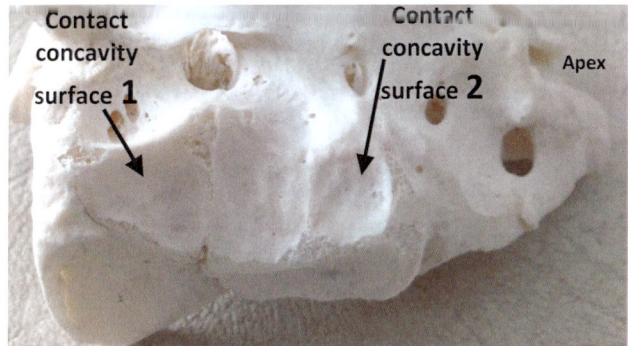

Figure P15D shows the superior surface of a sacrum. The indented concavity contact surfaces 1 and 2 are where the sacrum is forced against the triangle. .

The Bony mass has a triangle inferiorly

The iliac bony mass has a dividing triangle at its inferior border. It is situated above the "E"iliac facets. This is shown in **figures P15A** & **P15B**. It is an important safety feature to block excessive weight bearing placed on the "F" and "D" facets. If it was not for this triangle excessive weight and side-shift would buckle the pelvis and cause it to collapse.

Figure P15C, shows the side of a sacrum to illustrate the 'Prvy' bony area above the facets.

Figure P15D, is a photo of the sacral posterior surface showing contact surfaces that meet the sides of the bony triangle. These are important areas to be aware of.

Weight bearing rotation

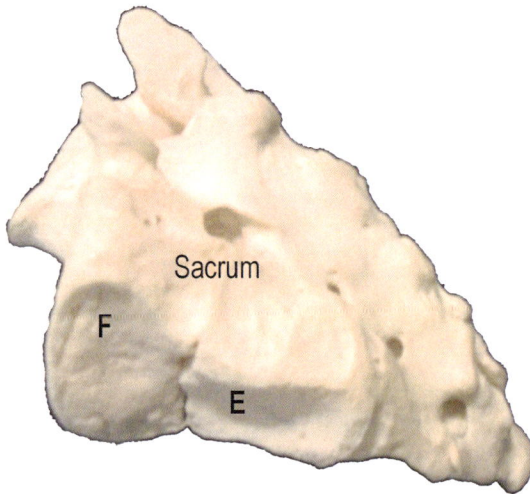

Figure P16A is a photograph of the sacral facet contours.

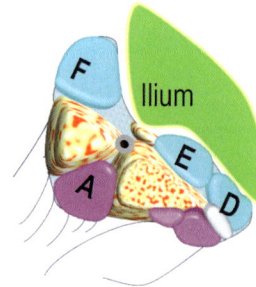

Figure P16B is an illustration of the iliac facet contours.

Pelvic rotation at the point of weight bearing

In the walking stride as body weight is transferred to one side, a local rotation takes place that rotates the whole pelvis to lever the leading leg into a straight path ahead.

How the pelvis rotates is determined by the shape of the Iliac facets as weight transfers from the 'E' facets to the 'F' facets. As Illustrated in **figures P16A and P16B**.

With the aid of the 'A' facet angle the leading leg stays in the mid-line. See **figures P10A and P10B**.

Look at the illustrations above, note that sacral facet 'E' bulges laterally. (Not all 'E' facets are as obvious as this real sacrum) but they nevertheless follow the same principle. This what makes peoples gaits different.

When weight direction transfers from the 'E' facet to the 'F' facet the full body's weight levers the symphysis pubis and lift the leading non weight bearing leg on the other side.

Crossover points

Figure P16C shows a photograph of a sacral facet with the S/I joint factors we have deduced, added. For completeness, the dividing ridge that runs horizontally along the middle of the S/I facets has also been added.

Not all S/I facets are shaped exactly the same, some have more or less convexity than others and some have more or less concavity or a mixture of both. Every human has an individual gait.

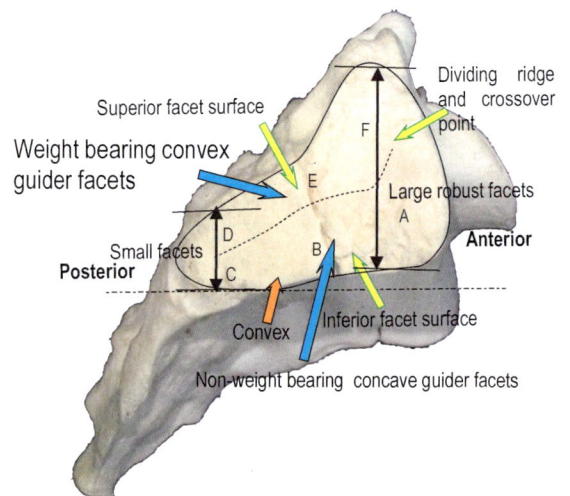

Figure P16C is a side-view of a sacral facet to illustrate the crossover points.

The mechanism that drives the sacroiliac joints

The driving force that causes the sacroiliac joints to articulate is rarely spoken about, if ever.

The first thing you notice about the sacroiliac joint facets is that they do not fit snugly together. The S/I joints are incorrectly presumed to be sliding joints when they are "elongated contact joints".

The sacral facets are held tightly against the iliac facets by a web of very strong ligaments. The ligaments have to be strong to allow the sacral facets to articulate with the iliac facets while weight bearing passes through.

With spinal weight bearing down and passing through the sacroiliac facets it would require an enormous amount energy to create enough direct force to drive any form of sacroiliac articulation.

If the sacroiliac articulations were muscle driven, we would expect to see some seriously strong small muscles but there aren't any.

Figures P17 A and **P17B**, show all the sacral muscle attachments and none of these muscles would be capable of providing the direction and power needed to articulate any form of sacroiliac articulation. It can therefore be concluded that the energy needed to drive the S/I joints is coming from another source.

We need to look for an energy source that is more powerful than the sum of the body weight bearing down on the base of the sacrum, with the ability to make the minute adjustments needed for articulation.

The answer to this riddle is simple. It is weight itself, or rather the distribution of weight. When body weight bears down it encounters an equal upward ground resistance known as the 'reactive force' travelling back up the legs. This meeting of opposing forces occurs at every cell in the body.

If a person stands on two legs, body weight is divided by the pelvis and transferred equally through each leg. If the person transfers their body weight to one side of their pelvis, the single leg on that side bears the full weight of the body.

However, it is physiologically impossible to transfer weight to one leg without side-shifting the pelvis towards the weight bearing leg. Without the side-shift the person would fall over.

Body weight and ground resistance collide at this pelvis and equal each other out. Therefore, it would take very little energy to lever the pelvis laterally under weight bearing conditions against an uneven facet surface. This makes pelvic side-shift a very powerful and efficient driving force.

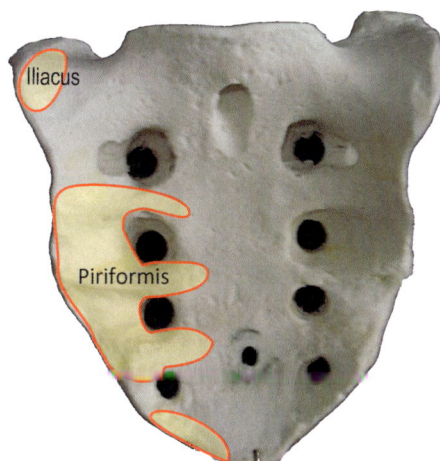

Figure P17A
Anterior view of sacral muscle attachments

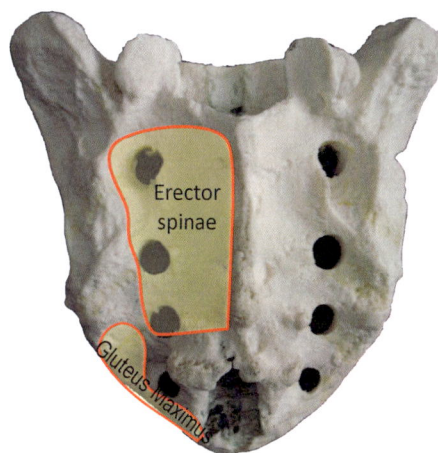

Figure P17B
Posterior view of sacral muscle attachments

Pelvic side-shift blocking

The dilemma facing pelvic side-shift is not so much about the mechanism needed to push it laterally, because the energy needed would be minimal. It is about the mechanism needed to block the side-shift from going too far. It is also about returning the pelvis to the midline.

Figure P18A is a stick view of the spine, pelvis and legs. The muscles etc. are represented in blue and the gravity forces in red-yellow arrows. The muscle and gravitational forces are all equal. This keeps the body in the midline.

If the pelvic muscles on the right in **figure P18B** relax and those on the left remain tight, this would generate enough muscle energy to side-shift the pelvis to the left.

See **figure P18C**. The strong quadrates lumborum muscles reside above the pelvis. They originate along the iliac crests and insert along the inferior posterior border of the twelfth ribs and the posterior lateral surfaces of the transverse processes of the upper four vertebrae. The angles of the tendons would allow this powerful muscle to graduate pelvic side-shift.

See **figure P18D**. Below the pelvis, the forces created by pelvic side-shift are greater than in the lumbar because of body-weight factors. Therefore, resistance to the pelvic side-shift requires more blocking power. This comes in the form of the strong elastic Iliotibial Tract and its tension governing muscle, the Tensor Fasciae Latae. The Gluteal and Piriformis muscles may also have a part to play in this process. The Iliotibial Tract is a strong fibrous sheath that acts as a strap that runs down the side of each thigh and graduates the side-shift to avoid jolts, and with the Tenser Fasciae Latae muscle, limits the amount of side-shift. The iliotibial tract originates from the Ilium and terminates at the lateral knee. It is generally considered by some as a knee stabilizer. During side-shift it becomes stretched. This elastic stretch helps to spring the pelvis back towards the midline or other side.

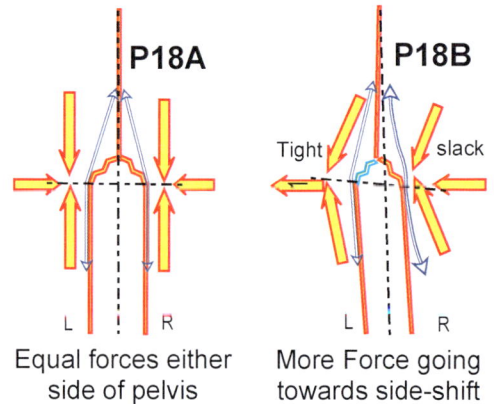

P18A

L   R

Equal forces either side of pelvis

P18B

Tight   slack

L   R

More Force going towards side-shift

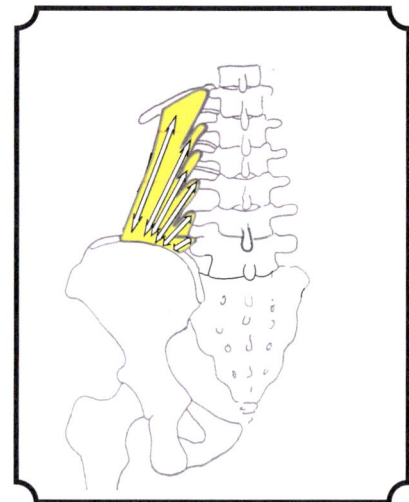

Figure P18C Posterior view of Quadratus Lumborum Muscle

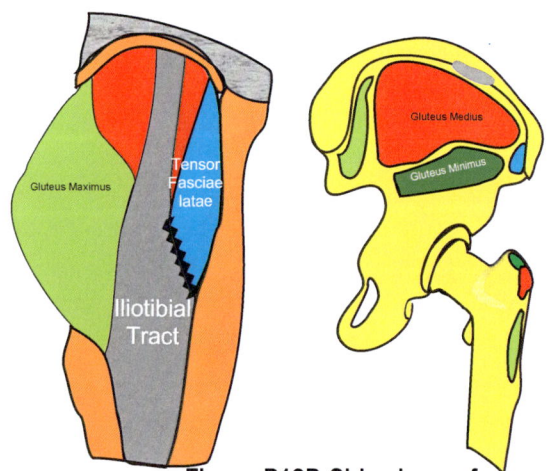

Gluteus Maximus

Tensor Fasciae latae

Iliotibial Tract

Gluteus Medius

Gluteus Minimus

Figure P18D Side views of Iliotibial Tract and Tensor Fasciae Latae muscle

18

Purpose of the long sacroiliac ligaments

When the pelvic ligaments are observed it can be seen that there are two long posterior ligaments on either side of the pelvis:

The sacrotuberous ligament, see **figure P19A**, attaches and anchors to the ischial tuberosity of the Ischial bone and stretches to the lateral sides of the sacrum and coccyx and lap over the sacrum as far as the spines. There is also a part that goes from the ischial tuberosity to the PSIS.

Figure P19B for completeness shows the short and strong posterior S/I ligaments.

The second long ligament is the sacro-spinous ligament, see **figure P19C**, which attaches and anchors to the ischial spine and stretches under the sacrotuberous ligament to attach to the sides of the sacrum and coccyx.

From a mechanical point of view, a longer ligament would have more stretch than a shorter one.

Logically, the placement of a longer ligament would indicate that there is some kind of shock-absorbing mechanism taking place in this area of the sacrum. So why at the apex of the sacrum?

To absorb the weight of the side-shifted body would require some considerable strength and rigidity. A short thick ligament would be better suited to this task. Hence the thick sacro-dorsal ligaments that lace the joint.

Crossover points

There are two crossover points, one at the anterior end and one at the posterior end of the S/I joint. These are shown in **figure P16C.**

At the anterior facets, where one leg is posterior and fully weight bearing whilst the other is lifted in the air with the foot anterior. 'F' to 'A'

Posterior facets. The point where the leading leg is anterior and touches the ground and then becomes load bearing 'C' with the trailing leg taking equal weight 'D'. At this crossover point, without damping, the leading leg contact with the ground would be jerky or even jolt.

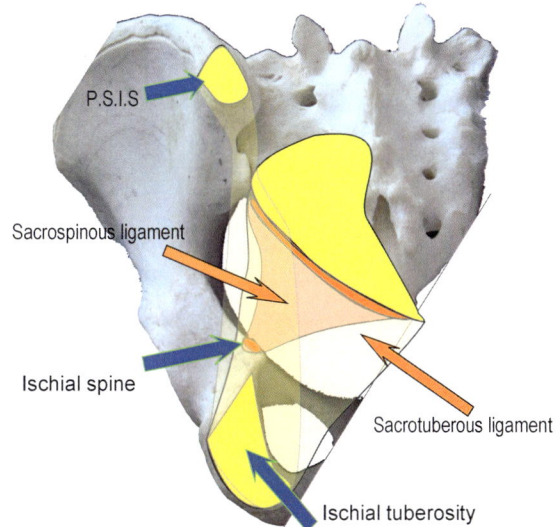

P.S.I.S

Sacrospinous ligament

Ischial spine

Sacrotuberous ligament

Ischial tuberosity

Figure P19A Posterior view of the long sacral ligaments

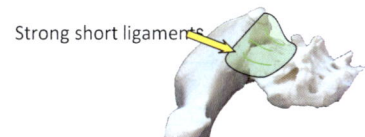

Strong short ligaments

Figure P19B Posterior view of the S/I posterior ligaments

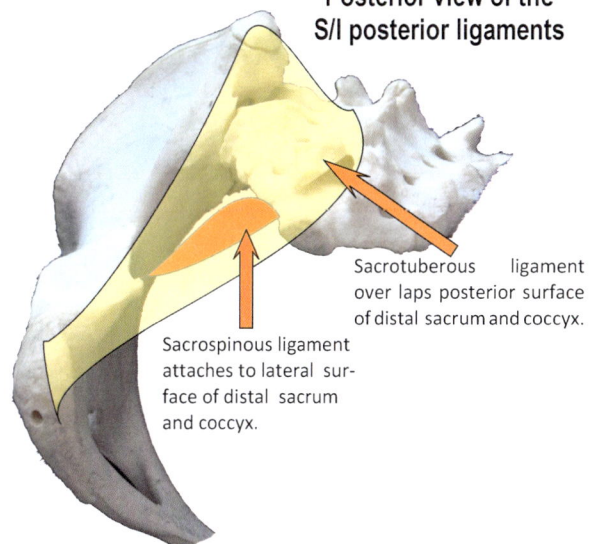

Sacrotuberous ligament over laps posterior surface of distal sacrum and coccyx.

Sacrospinous ligament attaches to lateral surface of distal sacrum and coccyx.

Figure P19C Position of ligaments seen from underneath pelvis

The mechanics behind the long sacroiliac ligaments

The shock absorbers of the pelvis

The S/I joints are encased in strong ligaments to bind them tightly together. Their job and along with the symphysis pubic ligament is to hold the joints steady and limit local movement.

Figure P20C, shows one side the Sacrospinous and Sacrotuberous ligaments that are positioned on either side of the sacrum. They act as shock absorbers to remove any jerking movements during weight bearing activities like ambulation.

The main times of maximum strain are shown in **figures P20A** and **P20B**.

These ligaments also cushion the swivel that takes place between the "E" to "F" and "A" to "B" facets. See **figure P10B**.

The long ligaments have more flexibly to pull and dampen the transitional rotations that take place.

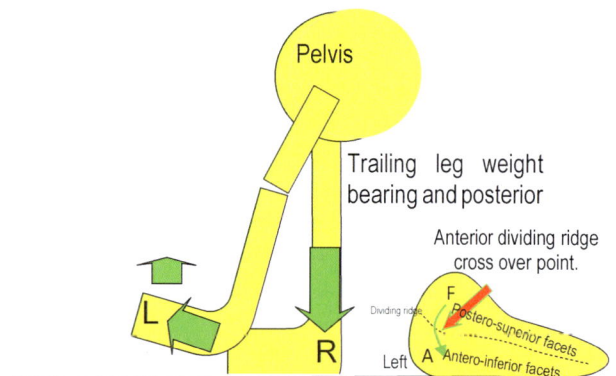

Figure P20A Anterior cross over point during walking

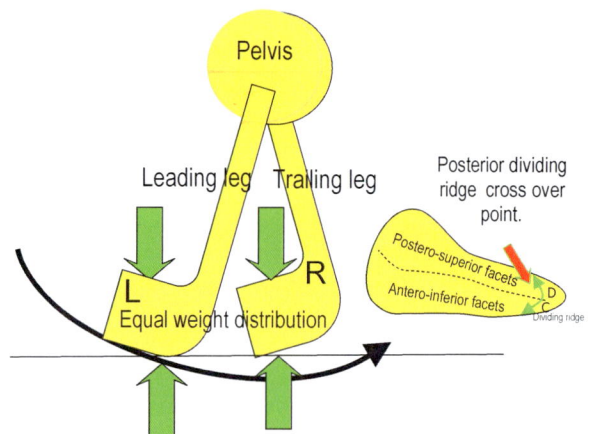

Figure P20B Posterior cross over point during walking

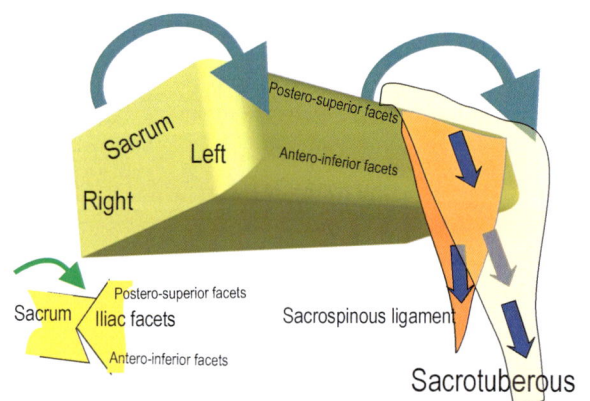

Figure P20C The Sacroiliac superio-posterior facets are brought together by long ligaments.

20

Theoretical load bearing stresses placed on the innominate bones

The pelvis is a complicated bony structure and clearly it is not entirely feasible to represent the forces therein by analogy to simple structures such as beams or frames. However, if the pelvis is seen as a beam, with the acting downward force (bodyweight) vertical at mid span and reactions vertically upwards at each end (femurs acting as struts), connections being 'ball joints' let into the beam, then the forces would be as shown in **figure P21A**.

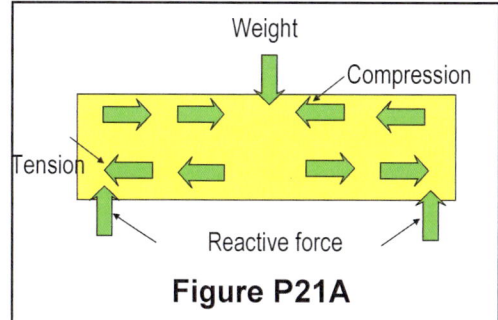

Figure P21A

There would be local forces in the ends of the beam in the form of a stress bubble as shown in **figure P21B**.

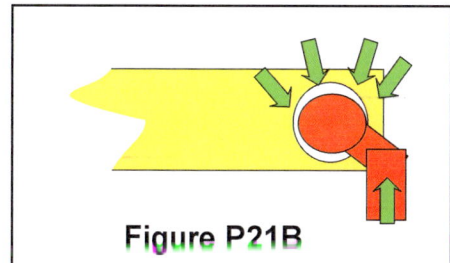

Figure P21B

If the pelvis was to be seen as a simple frame with the same actions and reactions, there would be both tension and compression in different parts of the structure, as shown in **figure P21C**.

For a joint to remain static, all forces must balance. If, for example, mainly downward force is not vertical but can only be supported vertically (a femur in an upright position), then there must be a balancing force somewhere, a triangle of forces applies as shown in **figure P21D.**

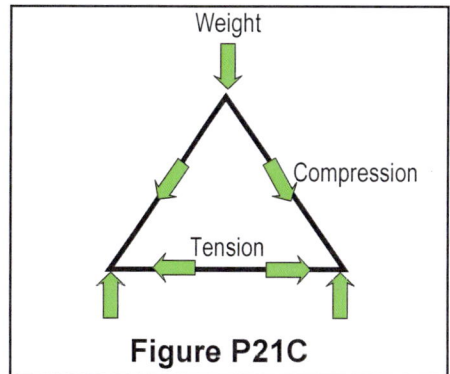

Figure P21C

And if this was to be applied to one side of the pelvis there would be tension, as shown in **figure P21E.**

It is suggested that, as the pelvis is not a simple structure, the forces would look something like those shown in **figure P21F.**

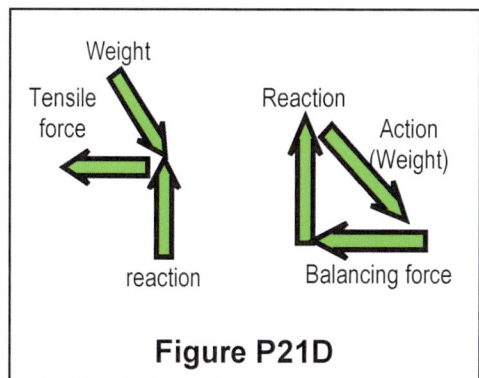

FigurP21E

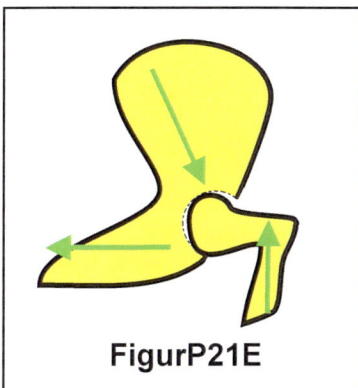

Figure P21F

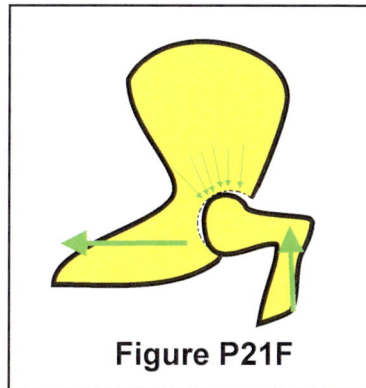

Figure P21D

Point of pivot

Weight bearing forces travelling down the lumbar spine arrive at an angle when they link with the base of the sacrum. See **figure P22B**.

From **figure P22A** it can be seen that the flexed shape of the lumbar spine acts much like a spring. It flexes when weight is bounced through it, typically when a person is walking. This softens the impact on the S/I joints.

Figure P22C is a photograph of the underside of a sacrum. Note that the tapered sides of the sacral facets are wedge shaped and lodge against the reciprocally shaped iliac facets.

Figure P22D illustrates the point of pivot. This very important area is where the sacral facets pivot on the iliac facets. It is the hub of the sacroiliac/iliosacral joints and the axes that allow the sacral facets to move about the iliac facets and vice-versa.

When a person is stationary and standing upright, the point of pivot is where body weight passes through the iliosacral/sacroiliac joints. Such a point also allows for readiness of motion in any direction.

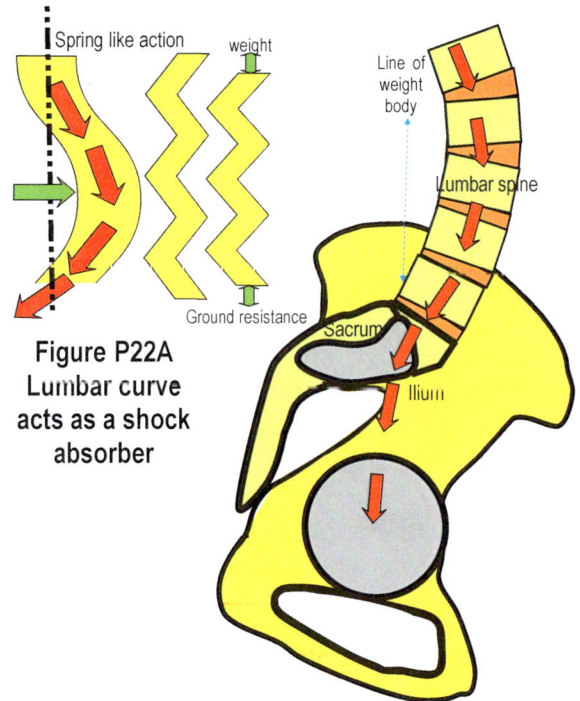

Figure P22A
Lumbar curve acts as a shock absorber

Figure P22B
Illustrating how weight is absorbed and distributed

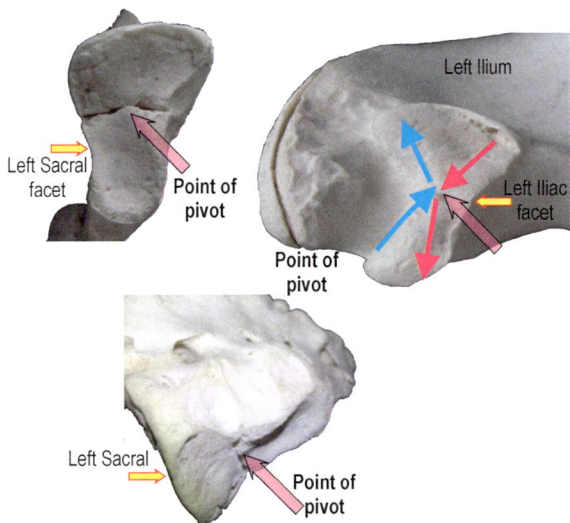

Figure P22D
Illustrates the pivot point from which all sacroiliac and iliosacral movements emanate when standing in the midline with equal weight bearing

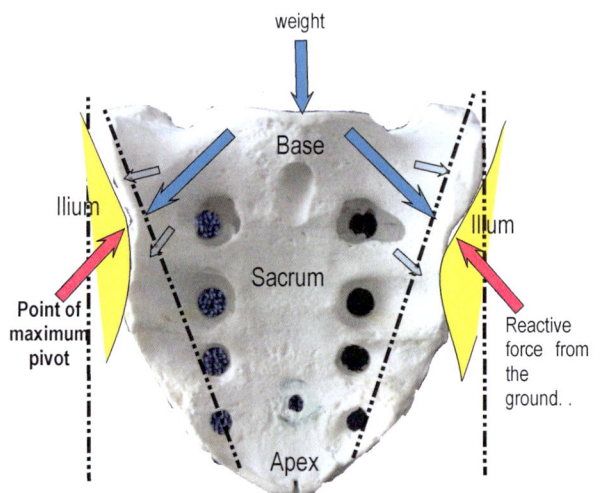

Figure P22C
Illustrates the blocking wedge shape of the sacral facets

Chapter Two
Pelvic lesions

Pelvic lesion

Figure P23, is a photo of a woman with the L3 R-R lesion pattern. As you can see her pelvis veers to the right. This is a typical pelvic lesion and seen in many, including top actors and sports people.

Her pelvis is superior and anterior on the right. This combination causes her right leg to rotate left and angle medially as it approaches the knee.

The left lower cheek of her bottom is posterior and lowered and twisted. Though not seen in this photo, her left foot is rotated laterally, and the right medially. You'll see this often.

The misaligned position of her pelvis due to gravity is reflected in her spine and shoulder girdle.

The question has to be asked, how the minute lesioned S/I joints cause such a huge misalignment of the body?

This misalignment within her gait will most likely cause restrictive movements, and hasten degenerative changes in the articulation of her legs, spine, shoulders, and ribs.

Such a general misalignment will ultimately put stress on all the joints of the body and increase the likelihood of arthritis, which is a wear and tear disorder.

Most Osteopaths and Chiropractors talk of correcting the sacroiliac/iliosacral joints. They never talk about the underlying self-reinforcing pelvic lesion that locks-in the sacroiliac/iliosacral lesions.

If the pelvic lesion is not addressed, corrected sacroiliac and iliosacral lesions will reappear on weight bearing.

Classical manipulation will help patients to get out of back pain, but commonly used manipulations will not correct the underlying pelvic lesion.

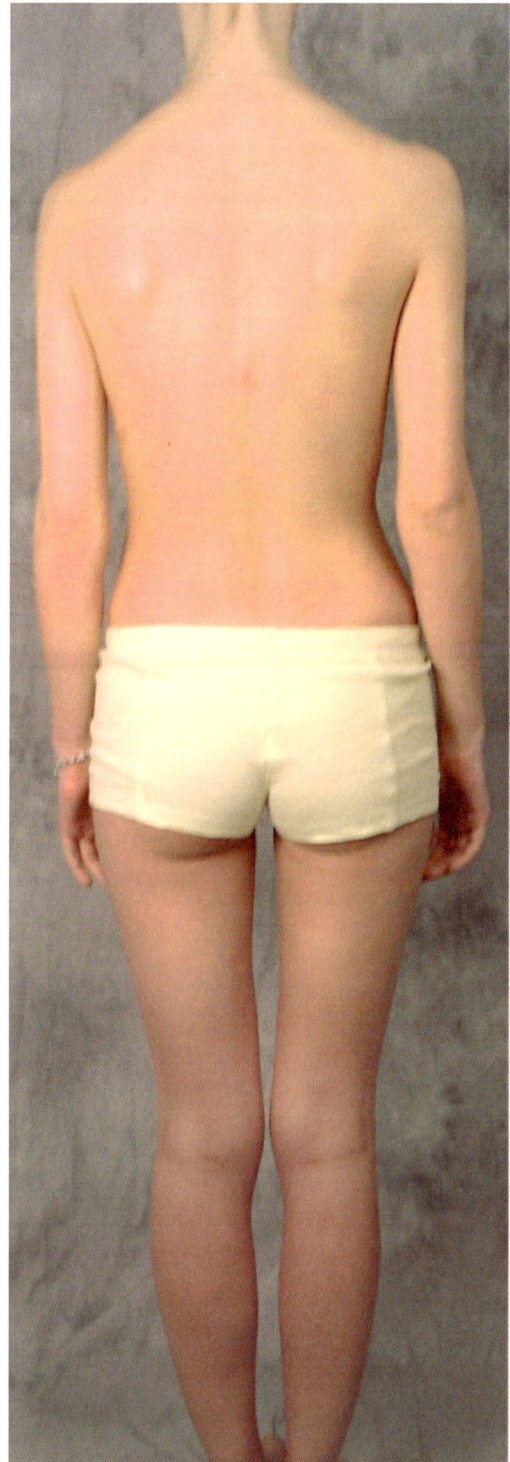

Figure P23 how a Pelvic lesion presents

Research: Sacroiliac imaging

On the previous chapter we deduced the type of axes the sacroiliac facets would need to function efficiently and the source of the huge amount of energy that would be required to generate movement. It is therefore time to take a step back and look at some of the introspective research that has been undertaken in recent years using highly accurate imaging technology and see how their results might fit in.

Wang and Dumas determined that the sacrum articulated around an orthogonal Axes. These axes are illustrated in **figure P24A**. Orthogonal in mathematical terms means two lines at right angles to each other. However, as you can see this does not apply to the **Y**, y axes.

In illustration, **figure P24A**, using axes 'X' as an example, the primary axis of movement is shown by the larger red arrow 'X' = superio-inferior, and the minor axis of movement by the smaller red arrow 'x' = lateral-lateral. In summary, the forces at work cause the sacrum to move in a superio-inferior direction whilst moving marginally to the left and right.

With the use of tantalum metal markers *Sturesson et al* used highly accurate Roentgen Stereophotogrammetric Analysis (RSA) to assess sacroiliac facet articulation. Their findings suggested that 1.3 degrees of rotation took place around a 3D helical screwing axis. Of this, 90% of the movement was recorded around the **X** axis, vaguely described as 'nutation' (nodding). The 'nutation' theory was originally recorded by *Weisl*. The other 10% axes were responsible for the magnitude of rotation and their translation and were represented by the addition of the x, **Y**, Y and **Z,** z axes.

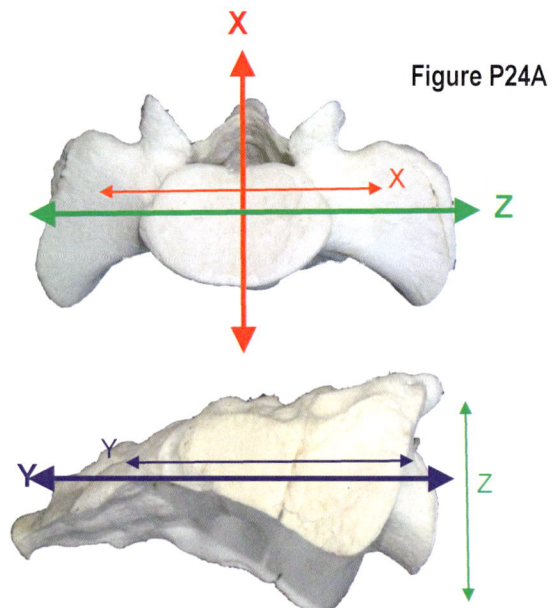

Figure P24A

Anterior and side-views of Sacrum
Wang M, Dumas GA determined the presence of XYZ Orthogonal Axes. Prime axes are shown in bolder lines and their minor axes are shown in thinner lines.

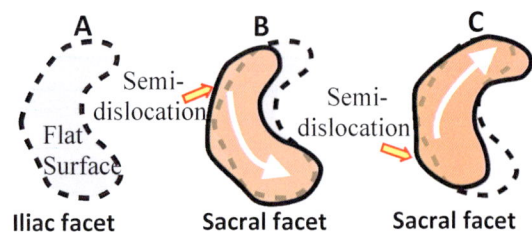

Figure P24B Nutation theory (as presented).

However, it was found that no two sacroiliac joints followed the exact same axes and varied from side to side. Other contemporary studies have found between 1- 2 degrees of articulation along the **X** axis, with a greater evolvement of the **Z** axis.

Sadly, this detailed research must have been performed on lesioned pelvises as it does not explain the normal human pelvic movement, though for some it confirmed the validity of the semi-dislocation 'nutation' theory see **figure P24B**. The above research explains the type of sacroiliac and iliosacral lesions found in a lesioned pelvis, for that, it must be commended.

The sacroiliac dividing ridge

No two sacroiliac facets are identical. In some, the surfaces are clearly defined and in others, they are almost flat. However, they all share the consistent characteristic ridge running like a rail along the middle that divides the facet into two halves. In the iliac facet shown in **figure P25A**, the ridge is well defined.

Axes **X**, x and **Z**, z in **figure P24A** are identical, though each places a different emphasis on their major and minor movements. This would indicate that there are two distinct axes in play.

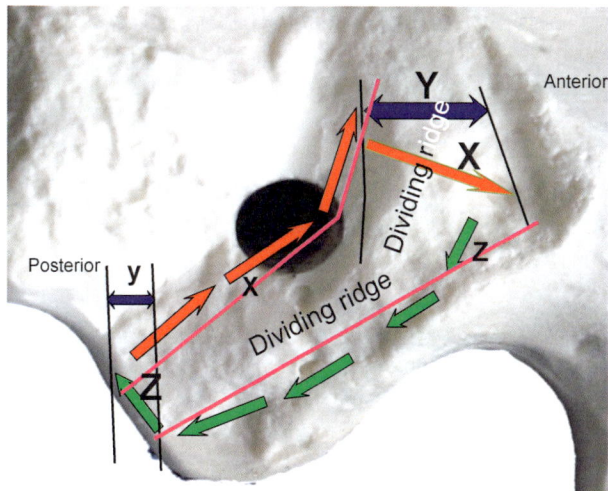

Figure P25A is a view of facets showing the cross over points

We know from **figure P24B** that movement takes place along horizontal axes during ambulation. The elongated axes that the facets follow require a method of returning to their starting position without incurring a head-on collision with the facets returning the other way, as one leg moves forward and the other stays still. The most efficient way to do this would be to divide the two facet surfaces with a middle ridge/island, so that the two way traffic is separated and able to flow in opposite directions.

At the anterior and posterior ends of the sacroiliac facets the dividing ridge would have to be crossed. The most obvious way to do this without dislocating the joint would be to rock the facets over the ridge in a kind of see-saw action, see **figure P26B.** If the sacrum were to slide over the perimeter edge, it would semi-dislocate the joint. See **figure P25B**.

The angle and distance at the crossover is very different at either end of the facets and accounts for several of the different axes. In **figures P25A** and **P25B**, the superio-inferior 'X, x' axes are illustrated by the red arrows**.** The minor superio-inferior '**Z**, z' axes by the green arrows. The major and minor anterio-posterior '**Y**, y' axes by the purple arrows. The lateral axes needs to be viewed from different angles.

Sacral Axis	Major Movement	Minor Movement
X, x	**Supero-inferior**	Lateral left-right
Y, y	Antero-posterior	Antero-posterior
Z, z	**Lateral left-right**	Supero-inferior

Figure P25B
Chart showing summary of researched sacroiliac articulation.

How translation occurs

Figure P26A illustrates three different boxed views of the sacrum.

A1 Shows the sacrum in neutral. **B1** with left side rotation superior, and **C1** with the right side rotation superior.

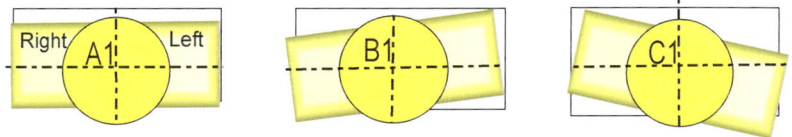

Figure P26A is an anterior view of the base of the sacrum as it rotates and side shifts from side to side.

If we were able to observe the sacrum performing these axes of rotation in cross section, it would be seen that the sacrum moves marginally from side to side. This would account for the **Z** and x axes. Viewed from the side, this same action would account for the superio-inferior **X** and z axes. Greater discrepancies would be seen in lesioned joints.

The base view illustrations in **figure P26A** B1 and C1 show how the sides of the sacrum tilt along this mid-line axis. With reference to the red and green arrows illustrated in **figureP25A** on the previous page, it is not hard to envisage how these crossover points would fit in.

The more angled dividing ridge, is the more pronounced at the anterior end than at the posterior end. This would explain the difference in the minor x lateral right-left and the **Z** major lateral right-left axes. When all these axes are added together a number of transla-tion movements occur simultaneously and or in series, depending on which part of the cycle the joint is at, at the time.

Figure P26B illustrates the rocking mechanism that makes it possible for the facet crossover to take place. The two crossover points differ in both angle and size of movement. Together with the concave and convex facet surfaces on both sides working in opposite lanes, the working joint under microscope would appear to be constantly fluctuating with no apparent axes, especially when the facets on both sides were in lesion.

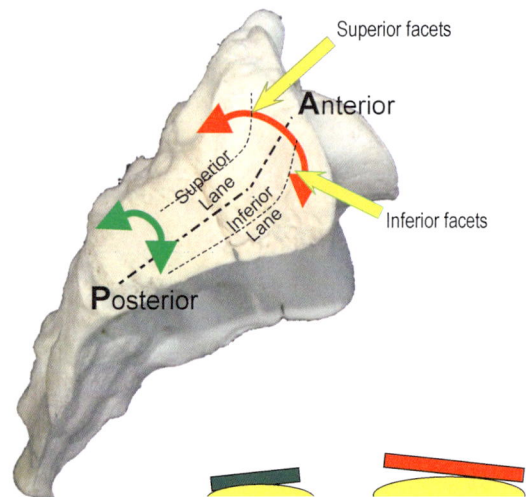

Figure P26B
Side-view of sacral facets illustrating how sacral articulation occurs in a healthy joint.

Sacroiliac facet subluxations

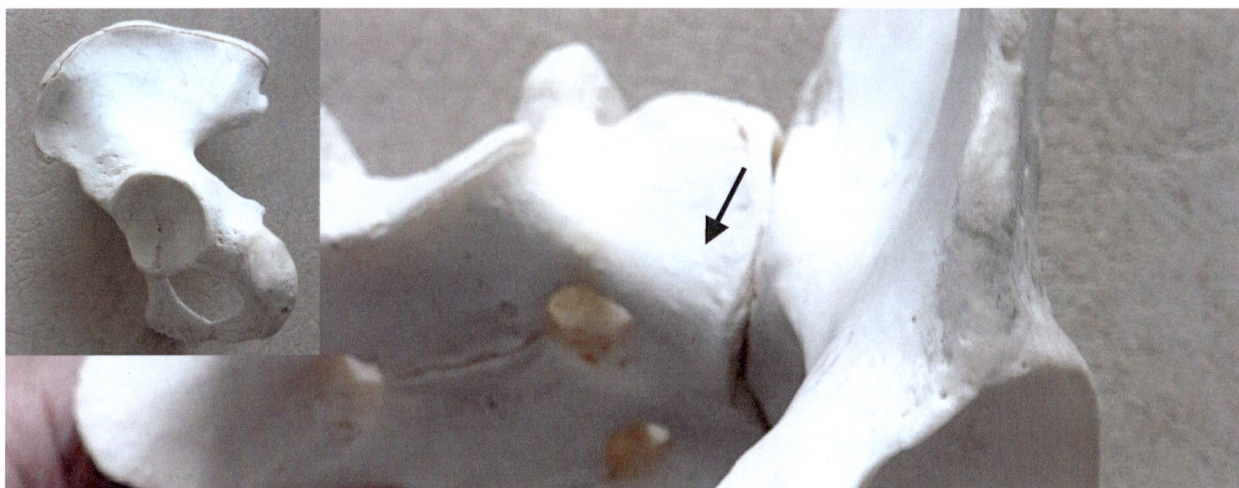

Figure P27A, Shows the sacroiliac facet in lesion with the Iliac facet, as per the research.

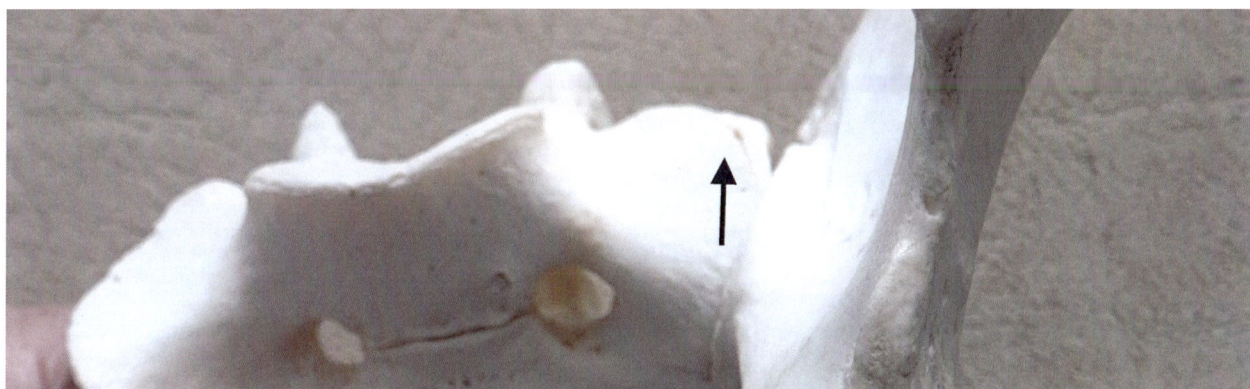

Figure P27B, shows the sacroiliac facet in lesion with the Iliac facet, as per the research.

Sacroiliac subluxations that lead to Osteopathic lesions.

Figure P27A, shows a sacral lesion where the sacral 'A' facet has been forced inferiorly on the iliac 'A' facet.

Figure P27B, shows a sacral lesion where the sacral 'F' facet has been forced superiorly on the iliac 'F' facet.

This is not normal articulation, this is lesioned/subluxated articulation.

It is hard to understand how these tiny displacement movements can turn into the Pelvic distortion seen in **figure P23.** That is because at the stage, pelvic side-shift and weight bearing have not been taken into account. When the positions of the facets, side-shift and weight bearing are taken into account, the dynamics of a pelvic lesion can be understood.

Sacroiliac principal of reciprocation

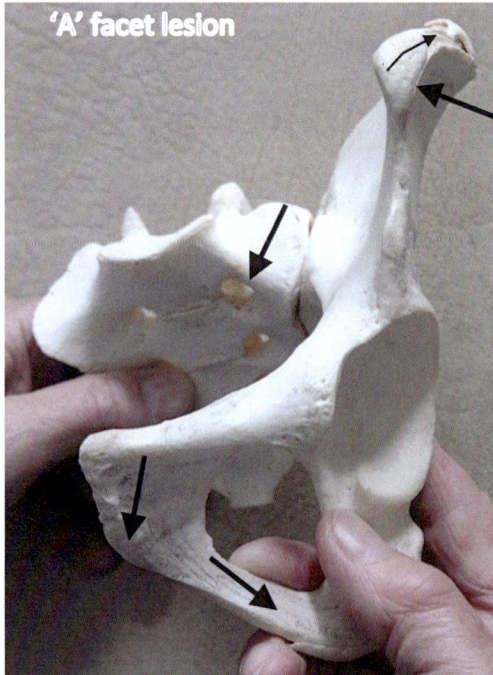

Figure P28A. Shows the direction of the lesioned 'A' facet

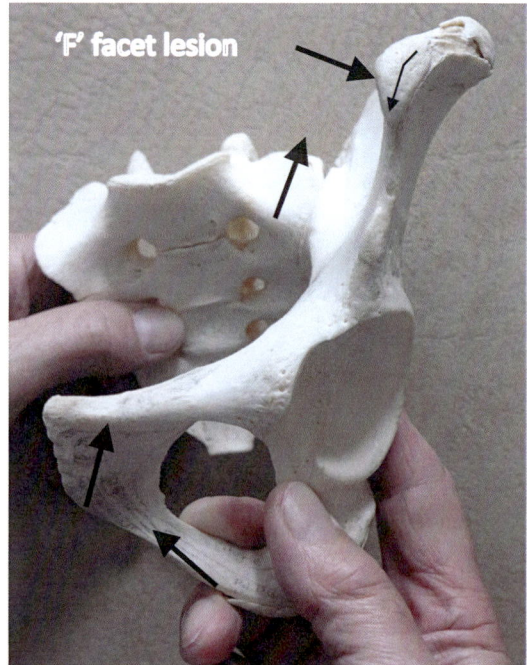

Figure P28C. Shows the direction of the lesioned 'F' facet.

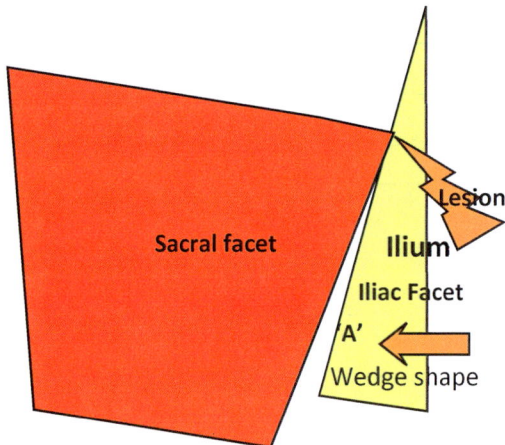

Figure P28B Shows where the lesioned 'A' facet gets caught against the wedge shaped side. See figure P12B.

These figures are self explanatory.

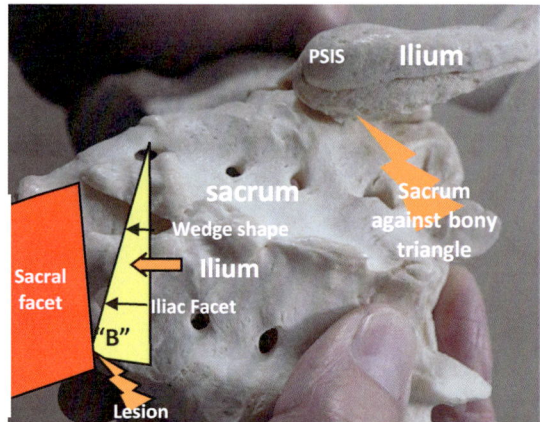

Figure P28D is a view from above showing where the 'F' lesioned sacrum presses against the bony mass triangle. The displaced sacral facet is levered over the border of the iliac facet between 'B' and 'C' area and gets trapped under the iliac 'B' facet. See crude illustration P24B,C. This what locks it in. See figure P14A.

Introduction to the beginning of pelvic Lesion

Pelvic lesion

Do not be confused by the old terminology used by Fryette. His theories were proved to be inaccurate in the 1980's by common sense and highly accurate imaging research.

From my book **"Advanced Osteopathic Technique"** we know that a sacroiliac and iliosacral lesion originate from the way L3 becomes lesioned. It has two choices. It can lesion with rotation to the right and side-bending to the right (L3 R-R), and side-bending to the left and rotation to the right (L3 L-R). These lesions create very different lesioning patterns in the body and are known for osteopathic purposes as R-R and L-R. The lady in **figure P23** is a R-R, which in the western world is the most common skeletal misalignment. This is the one we are going to concentrate on.

Most Osteopaths and Chiropractors routinely correct the sacroiliac and iliosacral lesions and L3 and L1 with hand me down marginally modified classical techniques that originated from the last century. They wrongly assume they are correcting the misalignment of the pelvis. They are not.

The problem for Osteopaths and Chiropractors in the R-R pelvic lesion pattern is that the original sacroiliac and iliosacral lesions that created the pelvic lesion, become locked in by the pelvic lesion. Once the pelvic lesion has been established, when reactive force returns up the legs, the whole pelvis is forced to distort further, and further lock-in the original sacroiliac and iliosacral lesions. The pelvic lesion is reinforced with every weight bearing step humans take.

Research has confirmed that corrected sacroiliac and iliosacral lesions when manipulated do not hold and return to their former lesioned position. Muscle based treatments attempting to correct a pelvic lesion in this respect are nonstarters. The following pages detail the process of why the subluxated sacroiliac and iliosacral joints cause self-reinforcing pelvic lesions.

Figure P29A, is an illustration of a normal pelvis as it was designed. The legs shown as arrows angle straight ahead.

Figure P29B, is an illustration of pelvic lesion. In the R-R lesion pattern, the legs shown as arrows are forced to go off at an angle. The lesioned pelvis reinforces these feet displacements with every walking step a human takes. Such a misalignment puts enormous strain on all the joints above and below. This can lead to premature arthritis.

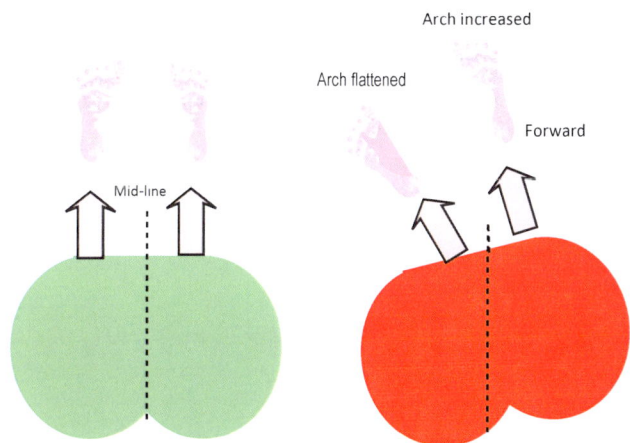

Figure P29A shows the non-lesioned pelvis. Legs aligned.

Figure P29B shows the misalignment a lesioned pelvis creates on the legs.

How the pelvis was designed to function normally during walking

Walking and the pelvis

When looking at the detailed angles of facets 'F' and 'A', it is easy to forget the wedge shape of the sacroiliac facets. **See figure P30A. Figures P7A** and **C** cover the unique shape and angles of the facets.

In **figure P30B,** it can be seen that the wedge shape plays and active role in directing the angles of the ilium and pubic bone.

To recap, from chapter one, the main rotation of the right ilium comes from the shape of the iliac facets between the 'E' and 'F' facets. See **figures P7A**, and **P10B**.

Function, when side shift is to the right. See figure P12B.

Right

Together with the shape and angle of the right 'F' facets, when pelvic side-shift is to the right, weight bearing is taken on the right leg, the iliac crest is forced laterally. This causes the right pubic bone to lift and swivel medially.

However, because the pelvic side-shift is to the right, the whole right side of the pelvis is pushed laterally away from the mid-line.

The weight bearing right acetabulum is pushed laterally. This pushes the femoral head and top of the femur laterally.

Left

The right lifted and rotated pubic bone lifts and angles the left pubic bone and draws the innominate medially.

When the left "A" facet is angled as per **figure P30B**, the left innominate angles more vertically and aims the left leg medially.

There comes a point where the right innominate can no longer side-shift to the right and blocks. The right full reactive body weight via the sacrum and pubic bone lifts the left innominate and angles the left leg forward. See **figure P30E**.

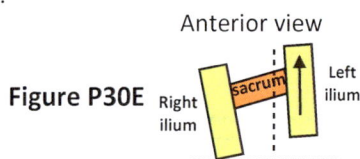

Figure P30A is a front view is an illustration of the wedge shape of how the sacrum in general mates with the Ilium

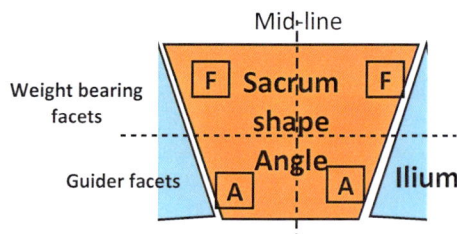

Figure P30B is a front view is an illustration of the wedge shape of how the sacrum in general mates with the Ilium

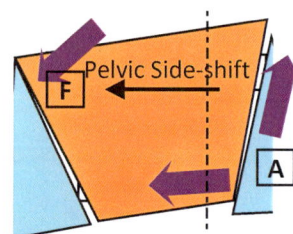

Figure P30D illustrates the normal right 'F' facet engaged with pelvic side-shift to the right.

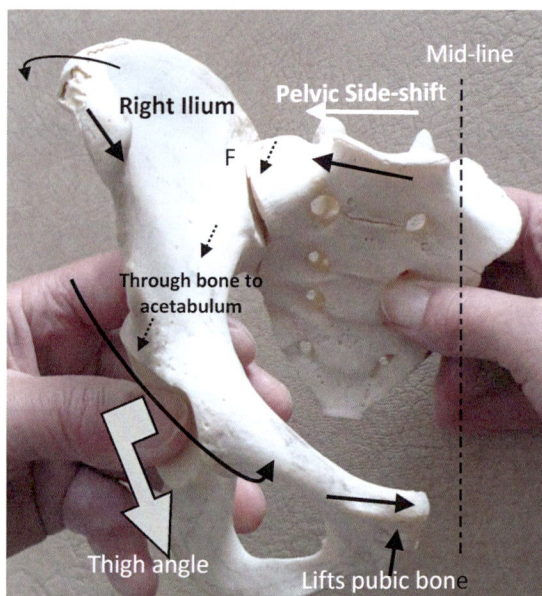

Anterior view

Figure P30E

30

How the pelvis malfunctions during walking to become the first stage of a pelvic Lesion

How the small misalignment of the "F" facet leads to a major problem.

Figure P31A, is an illustration of what was arrived at with the imaging research that is shown on **figure P24B**. You can see at the top, that subluxation shown in red, is posterior to the non-lesioned facet, shown in yellow. However, the area of most concern is the lesion between facets 'B' and 'C'.

Figure P29B. The 'F' facet lesion during side-shift right, causes the right iliac crest to lean laterally and further away from the mid-line. This causes the misaligned pubic bone to lift and rotate medially.

This lateral shift changes the placement of the points of force directed at the weight bearing right acetabulum and femoral head. This change is shown in **figure P31C** which changes the whole weight distribution placed on the right leg and creates a buckling effect. The outcome is that the right pubic bone angles further anteriorly, which projects the left innominate further forward. This displacement causes two major problems. The right leg is angled medially with a loss of stride length. The left leg is lifted and angled outwards with an increase of stride length.

Because the side-shift moves the right innominate further laterally and then eventually blocked at the triangle, see **figure P32D**, it forces the pubic bone away from the midline taking the left innominate closer to the right and further over the midline to affect the pelvic trajectory.

Figure P31D shows the angles of the innominates that result into:
Right foot = increased arch.
Left foot = dropped arch.

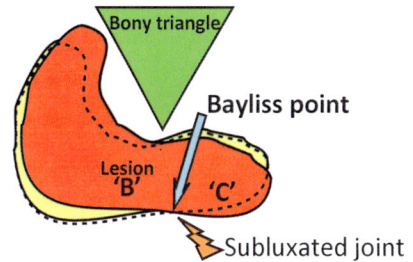

Figure P31A shows an "F" facet lesion. Yellow is correct position of the sacrum and red the misalignment.

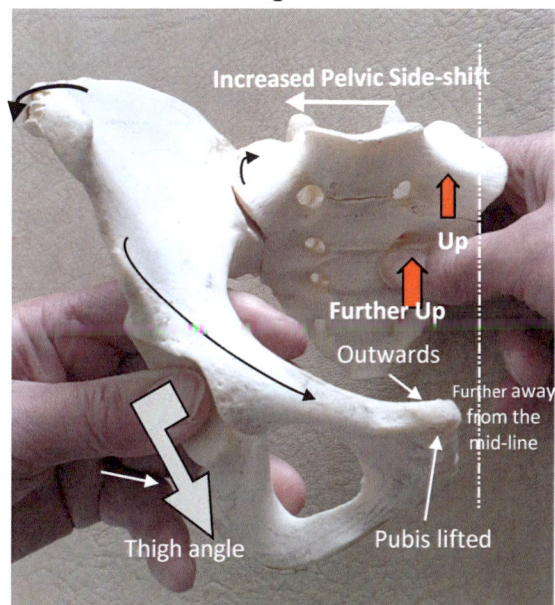

Figure P31B shows the iliac crest angled laterally which causes the pubic bone to lift and turn outwards in accordance with the 'F' facet lesion.

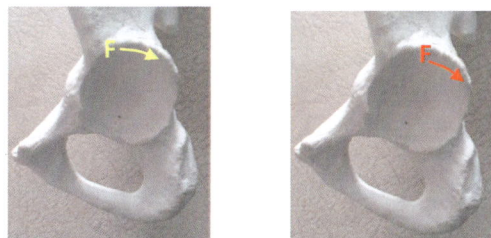

Figure P31C shows the weight displacement caused by the extra side-shift right and iliac crest flare.

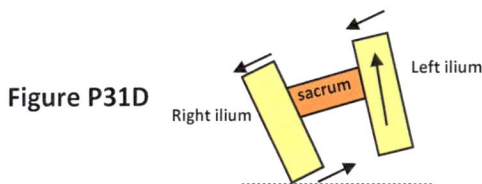

Figure P31D

Illustration showing position of the facets in the RR pelvic lesion part 1

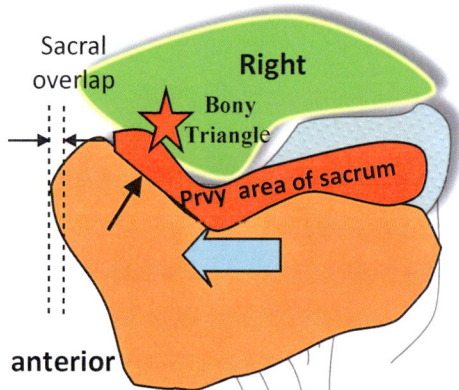

Figure P32A: is an exaggerated illustration of a right sacroiliac facet lesion in the RR pattern pelvis. Green is the iliac bony mass and the orange the sacral facet.

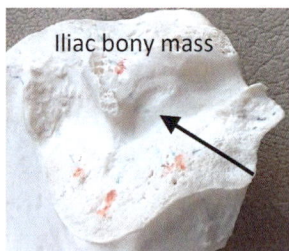

Figure P32E. Shows the slope of the posterior bony mass that forms the iliac triangle

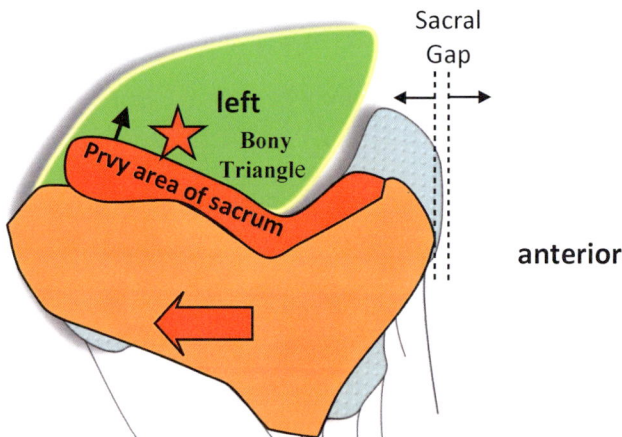

Figure P32C: is an exaggerated illustration of a left iliosacral facet lesion in the RR pattern pelvis. Green is the iliac bony mass and the orange the sacral facet. Due to the posterior slope of the ilium the sacral rides up the triangle.

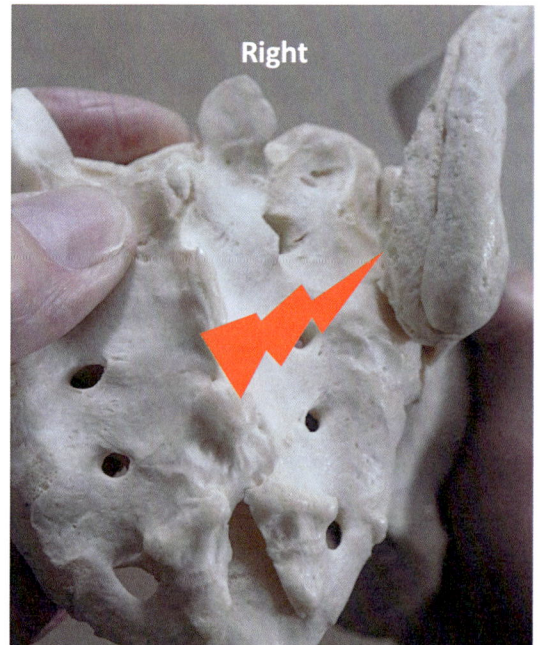

Figure P32B is a view from above showing the point of contact when the 'F' facet in lesioned as per figure P32A

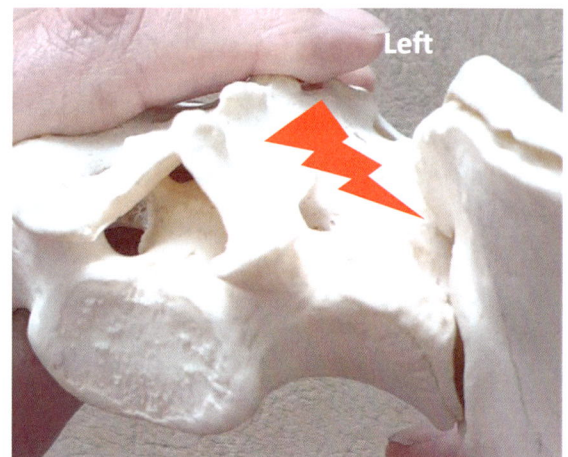

Figure P32D is a view from above showing an exaggerated view when the iliac lifts the 'D' facet away form the 'D' facet in the lesion shown in figure P32C. Also see Figure P28D.

Explanation showing position of the facets in the R-R lesion part 2

See page 32.

Figure P32A, is an illustration of the right sacroiliac facets in Osteopathic lesion. The red star indicates where the bone of the upper ridged surface of the sacrum (above the sacral 'F' facet meets with the bony triangle of the iliac bony mass.

Figure P32B, is a photo-illustration of the bone against bone from above the 'F' facet. This is very much a safety feature. When pelvic side-shift is to the right with in 'F' facet sacral lesion), see **figure P31B**, the right sacral 'F' facet joint begins to buckle and the ilium side-shifts further to the right. It would continue to side-shift right and dislocate if the Iliac bony triangle and iliotibial tract were not there to cushion and block the movement.

Figure P32C. This is where the pelvic lesion starts. It is important to know this. As it is catch 22.

The displacement of the lesioned sacral 'F' facet on the right, angles the left pubic bone incorrectly and alters the left facet alignment. In **figure P28B, P32D** and **E**, the sacrum has been guided by the pubic bone to force the posterior surface of the sacrum above the iliac 'D', against the left iliac bony triangle. Therefore, we have:

1) On the right, we have the posterior surface of the lesioned sacrum above the 'F' facet forced against the anterior iliac bony triangle. This is part of the pelvic lesion,

2) Also on the right, we have the sacral 'C' facet lesion wedged against the wedge shape of the iliac facet around the 'C' area.

3) On the right, we have the displaced right pubic bone transmitting the reactive force of the weight bearing right innominate through to the left side.

4) On the left, we have the displaced reactive force coming from the right, above the 'E' and 'D' facets pushing the posterior surface of the left sacrum and forcing it against the left posterior iliac bony triangle. It is locked there by the displaced right side.

5) Also, on the left. We have the left lesioned sacral 'A' facet wedged against the left iliac 'A' facet.

6) When the weight and side-shift are directed to the locked left innominate as in walking, the left leg becomes weight bearing. In turn, the left reactive ground force is transmitted via the sacrum and pubic bone to the locked right side. This causes the posterior surface of the right side of the sacrum above the lesioned 'F' facet to be forced against the anterior surface on the iliac bony triangle.

7) When weight and side-shift return to the right, the right reactive force travelling up the right leg lifts the displaced locked left innominate and guides the left leg forward and outwards. This causes the instep of the left foot to drop.

8) With the right innominate crest turned outward. The right leg is turned inwards with the foot arched.

The right innominate lesion

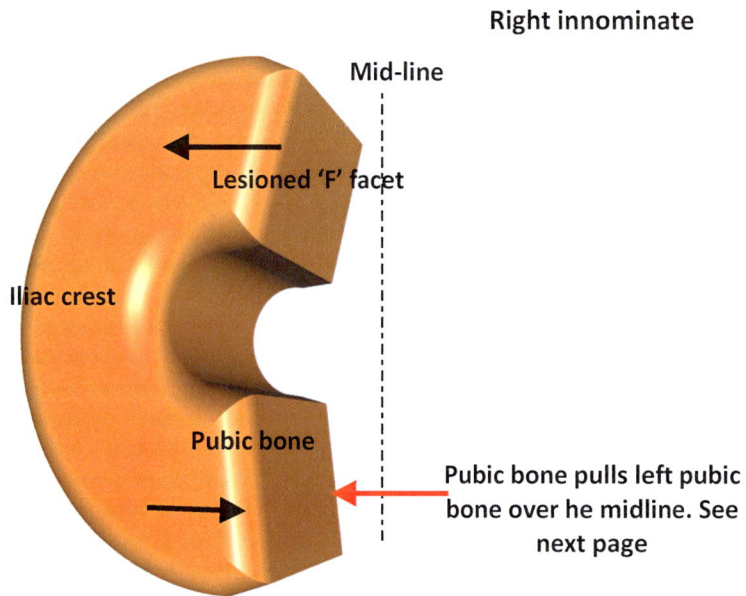

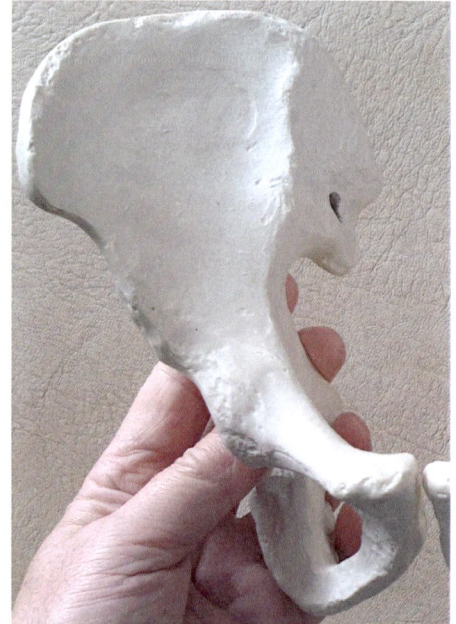

Right innominate

Figure P34A illustrates an anterior view of the the right innominate angle when the 'F' facet is lesioned. The innominate overly rotates and the iliac crest leans laterally and the right pubic bone and sacrum pull the left side innominate over the mid-line.

Figure P34B is an anterior photo of figure P34A to help make make the angles clearer.

R-R lesion on the right.

Figure P34A is an illustration of the right innominate in lesion due to an 'F' facet lesion on the right**.** When weight bearing, reactive forces travel up the displaced right leg and reinforce the rotation and lift the medial angle of the pubic bone.

The right leg is turned inwards and the right innominate remains to the right of the mid-line with the iliac crest fanned laterally.

The sacrum and pubic bone lift the left innominate higher than it should be and angle it laterally, so the left leg is turned outwards with a longer stride.

Figure P34B, for completeness, is a photo of a right innominate. It should make the illustration easier to understand.

The left A facet innominate lesion

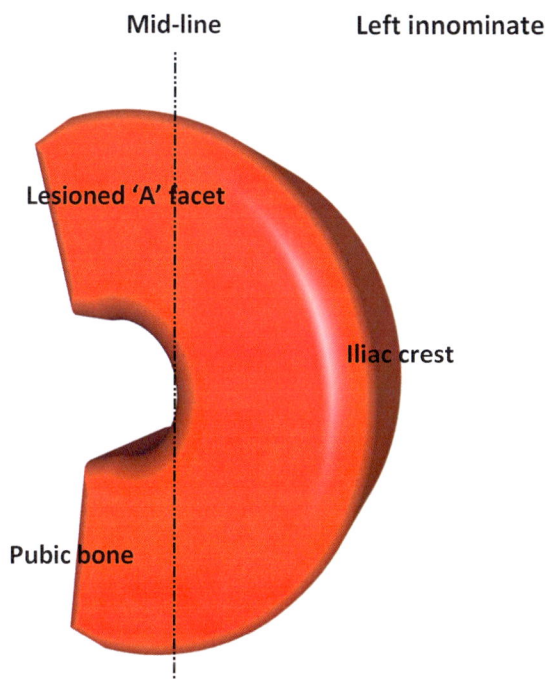

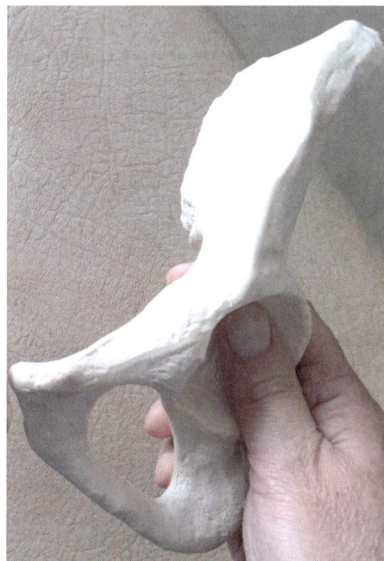

Mid-line   Left innominate

Lesioned 'A' facet

Iliac crest

Pubic bone

Figure P35A is an anterior view illustration showing the position of the left innominate when the sacral 'F' facet on the right is in lesion. It is dragged over the mid-line.

Figure P35B is an anterior photo of figure P35A to help make the angles clearer.

R-R lesion on the left when the right leg is weight bearing.

Figure P35A is an anterior illustration of the left innominate when the 'A' sacroiliac facet is dragged to the right by the lesioned right 'F' facet.

The right innominate via the pubic bone lifts the left innominate higher than it would be in its normal position and angles it laterally. This rotates the left leg laterally and the arch of the foot drops. With the additional height, the left leg stride becomes longer.

In normal articulation the left innominate would be more upright and leaning backwards.

Figure P35B is a photo of a right Innominate for completeness. It should make the illustration easier to understand.

Consequence of misaligned legs

When the left 'A' facet Iliosacral lesion is combined with the altered angles of the right pubic bone and sacrum, the following incorrect tracking angles take place.

To recap. The right sacroiliac lesion angled the left innominate higher than normal with the ASIS raised and turned it laterally instead of its correct medial direction.

Therefore, in turn, the left acetabulum lifts the left leg/foot further forward and laterally.

Figure P36A. As a consequence of the misaligned left innominate is that the walking stride follows a destructive trajectory. The lateral angle becomes exaggerated and obvious when reactive force travels up the left leg during walking. The left foot is turned outwards which drops the foot arch.

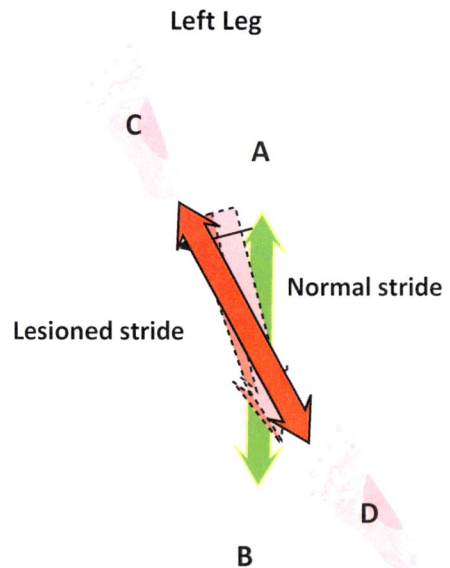

Figure P36A, illustrates the normal left leg trajectory labelled A-B in green, and the incorrect trajectory in red, C-D.

Figure P36B, illustrates the right leg/foot misalignment. The normal right leg trajectory is illustrated in brown. In the 'F' lesioned innominate the right ASIS dips inferiorly and shortens the stride at incorrect medial angle shown in blue. The right foot is angled inwards with an increased foot arch.

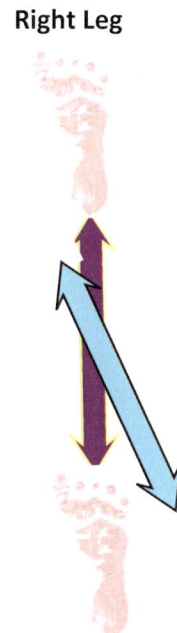

At this stage the foot placement is not what you the see when the R-R patient presents and stands in front of you. This is because further pelvic distortion is yet to take place.

Left Leg

Normal stride

Lesioned stride

C

A

D

B

Figure P36A shows the normal trajectory in green, and displaced trajectory in red.

Right Leg

Figure P36B shows the normal trajectory in brown and displaced trajectory in blue.

Misaligned left leg creates the R-R pelvic Lesion

The pelvic lesion locks in the sacroiliac and iliosacral lesions.

Brief recap:
The right innominate is lateral to the mid-line. The right 'F' facet sacroiliac lesion caused the right iliac crest to rotate and flare outwards. Via this misdirected force, the sacrum and pubic bone pull the left innominate medially in a clockwise rotation direction.

Figure P37A. The extra height forced on the left ilium angles the left leg further forward and at a lateral angle. At the same time the left foot is rotated clockwise. (Arch drops)

Figure 37B. As the weight bearing takes place under the misaligned left leg, and with the left 'A' facet in lesion engaged, the ilium is locked to the sacrum. The area above the 'D' facet at the bony triangle lifts left sacrum. The posterior sacral apex area is lifted in the direction of the misaligned left innominate. See **figures P32C** and **D**.

The reactive ground force that returns up the left innominate causes the posterior sacrum at the triangle to swivel the pelvis as a whole anticlockwise as per **figure P37A**.

Figure P37B, 1 and **2** are self-explanatory. The matchstick lines are illustrated to confirm the angles that take place in a R-R pelvis to establish the lesion.

Once the Pelvic lesion has established itself, it is reinforced with every step a human takes.

If the sacroiliac and iliosacral lesions are corrected before the pelvic lesion is corrected. They will return to their former lesioned position on weight bearing.

Key: *Like an arrow*

⊙ Towards you   ⊗ Away from you

view from above

Flat foot

Pelvis

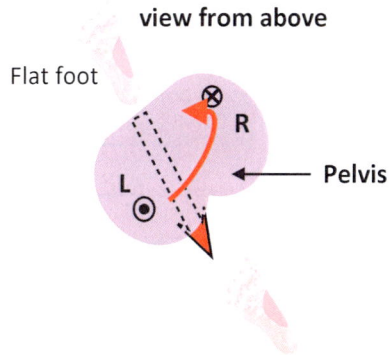

Figure P37A is an exaggerated illustration of the distorted swivel the outward left leg has on the pelvis.

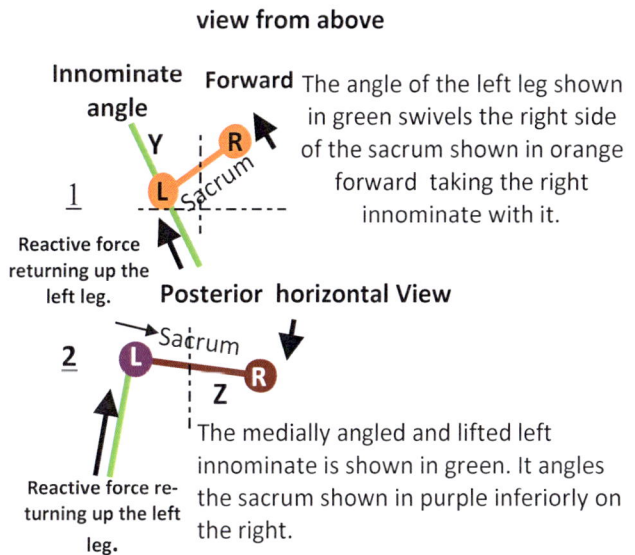

....

view from above

Innominate angle   Forward

The angle of the left leg shown in green swivels the right side of the sacrum shown in orange forward taking the right innominate with it.

Reactive force returning up the left leg.

Posterior horizontal View

The medially angled and lifted left innominate is shown in green. It angles the sacrum shown in purple inferiorly on the right.

Reactive force returning up the left leg.

Figure P37B is a matchstick illustration of the forces forced on the left side of the pelvis by reactive returning up the left leg. The green line is the left incorrect leg trajectory. The orange line is the angle forced on the left innominate. The purple line is the downward force passing through the sacrum on the right innominate.

The theoretical origin of the pelvic displacement in the R-R lesion pattern

The pelvic lesion

Over the past pages in this chapter, we have seen how a simple "F" facet lesion has turned out to permeate into a completely distorted pelvis. A pelvic lesion that is reinforced with every step a human takes.

At this stage, simply correcting the sacroiliac and iliosacral lesions with manipulation is no longer viable, as their corrected position will not hold on weight bearing.

Muscle techniques have no chance of correcting a pelvic lesion.

Following on from page 37, we see that the shape and function of the pelvis has radically changed. The whole body has lost its symmetry.

Figures P36A and **B** illustrate the displacement stage before the pelvic lesion takes place. The pelvic lesion changes the leg stride angles and placement.

Figure P38A. In the RR pelvic lesion, the right foot on standing with the feet together is anterior to the left foot. The left foot is turned out and the right turned in. This causes the human who walks straight ahead to walk like a crab. The crab pelvis.

Figure P38B. The illustration shows how the lesioned pelvis shown in orange is twisted and generally anterior on the right.

Figure P38A. Shows the exaggerated position of the feet during walking.

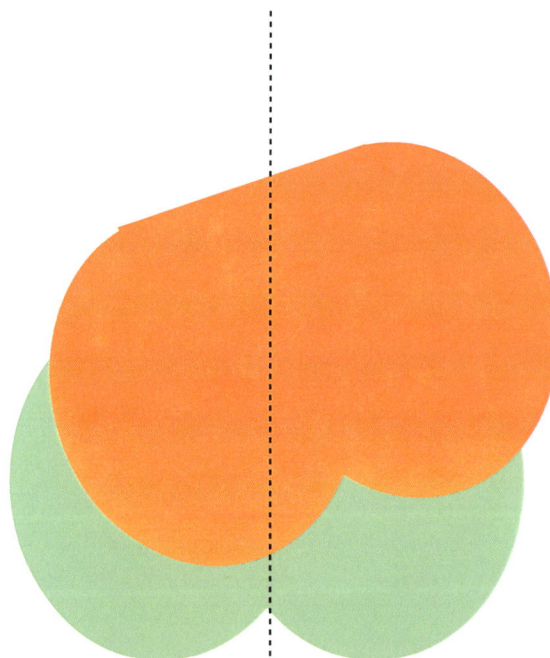

Figure P38B, is a view from above illustrating the displaced pelvic position in orange when weight bearing is taken on the left leg, compared to the correct position shown in green.

Pelvic lesion illustration in the R-R lesion pattern

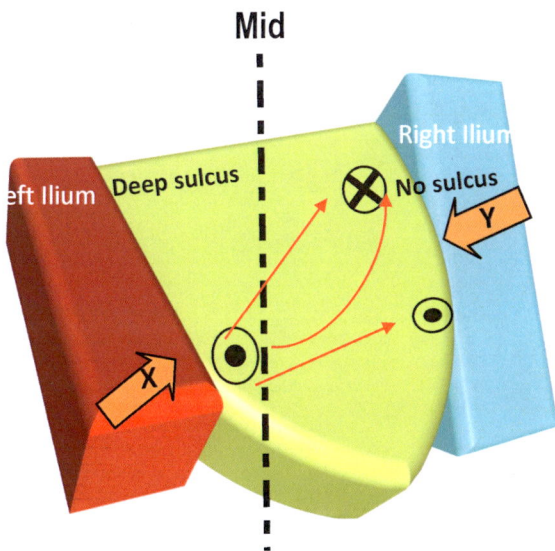

Mid

Left Ilium   Deep sulcus   Right Ilium   No sulcus

X   Y

Figure P39A. Showing the RR pattern iliosacral lesion on the left as patient presents.

Posterior ⬤   Anterior ⊗

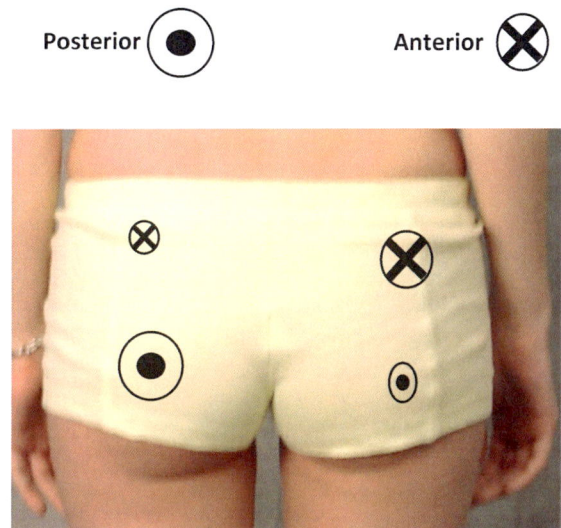

Figure P39B. Showing the RR pattern iliosacral lesion on the left as patient presents. Photo from page 23

Lesioned pelvis in the R-R pattern lesion.

Figure P39A. Is an illustration of a pelvic R-R lesion. The pelvis as a whole has been taken to the right side of body's   midline. The points of displaced facets are at the 'A' facet on the left iliosacral joint and the 'F' facet on the right sacroiliac joint. These lesioned joints at this point become trapped in by the pelvic lesion. Correcting the 'F' and 'A' facets will give some pain relief but will not correct the pelvic lesion which is reinforced every time the left leg becomes weight bearing. The result is that the corrected iliosacral and sacroiliac joints will be forced and levered back into lesion on weight bearing.

This observation is backed up by independent research that gave rise to a vocal professor. (His own BMA backed two research projects into alternative medicine were thrown out by the BMA and government as works of fiction). He claimed that there is no science in Osteopathy and Chiropractic. Both professions have proven through numerous patient surveys routinely that they get around 60-80% success rate in terms of getting patients backs out of pain and restoring varying amounts of mobility. However, because pelvic lesions are not recognised or taught, they are left untouched which means that every joint will go back out of place again on weight bearing. However, probably not in such a locked way.

Figure P39A, is an illustration of the areas of most concern: **X**, and **Y**. These two areas are where sacral contact is made with the bony triangle. As weight travels up the left leg, the areas of reactive force shown in orange, pass through the sacrum to the already displaced right ilium. See **figure P37B**.

Figure P39B, is a closer look at the pelvis of the lady on page 23. Look closely and you will see the shape of the illustration in **figure P39A** forced on her pelvis.

Consequences of pelvic lesion in the R-R lesion pattern: Torso

A pelvic lesion affects all the joints of the spine.

Figure P40A, is a photo of a slim lady with a R-R pelvic lesion. Because she is slim it makes it easier for us to see the problem areas in her back.

Take a long look at her back for a moment. Note the areas that would be of most treatment.

The area to look at after her pelvis is her shoulder girdle. You will see that her shoulders are a mirror image of her lesioned pelvis.

Her left shoulder has been forced away from the body's midline and angled anterior to match the right side of the pelvis in order to compensate and keep balance. Note the scapular is lower than the right.

Her right shoulder is raised and posterior. It has been forced over the body's mid-line to match the left side of her pelvis. Observe her right elbow.

All the lesions above the pelvis and below the shoulders are joints that have become compensatory. Correcting one or two of these joints will have no effect of straightening the pelvis.

The original L3 lumbar lesion is not easily identified, but it is there, and has become double locked-in by the compensating surrounding lumbar lesions.

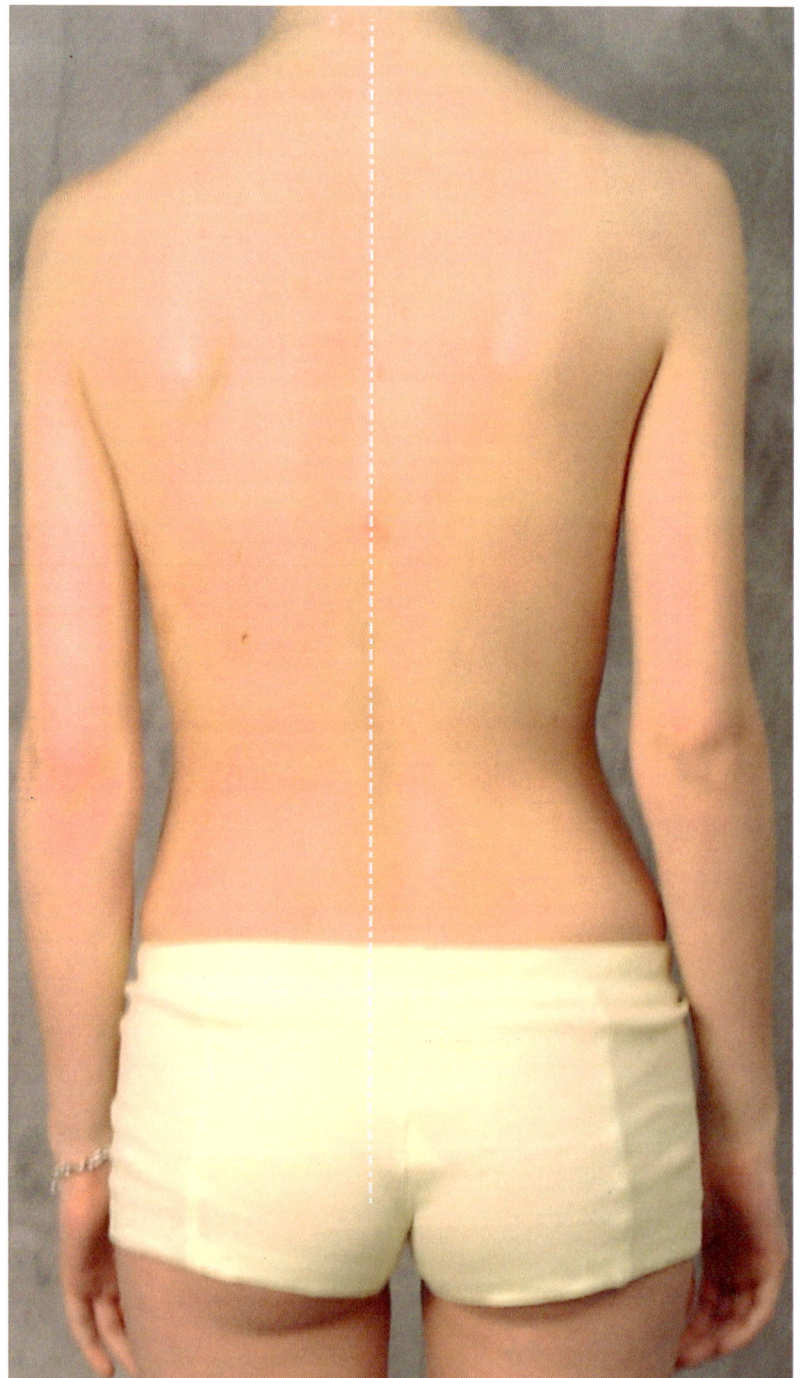

Figure P40A is a photo of the top half of the lady on page 23. This lady's back is misshapen by her pelvic lesion.

Consequences of pelvic lesion in the R-R lesion pattern: Hips and left leg

A pelvic lesion affects the alignment of the legs, spine, shoulders, and rib joints.

Figure P41A, is a photo of a slim lady with a R-R pelvic lesion. Because she is slim it makes it easier for us to identify her incorrectly aligned legs.

Take a long look at her buttocks, hip, knees, and legs. Note the area that you feel would be in need of correction.

In general, the left side of her pelvis is posterior and side-shifted over the body's mid-line to the right.

Left leg

The lower half of her left buttock is posterior.

Her left leg is angled laterally and can be confirmed by looking at the crease under her left buttock.

Her left leg is flexed at the knee.

Weight bearing on the inverted lateral angle of her left thigh bears down at on distal end of the femur where it meets the knee joint.

When weight bearing reactive ground force return up, through the left foot, the tibia at its meeting with the underside of the left knee puts an extra inverted force under the knee. This creates a screwing tension that can be seen in her left calf. This weakens the knee joint.

This same screwing action is passed on up to the hip joint.

This hip misalignment will affect its relationship with the Pelvis.

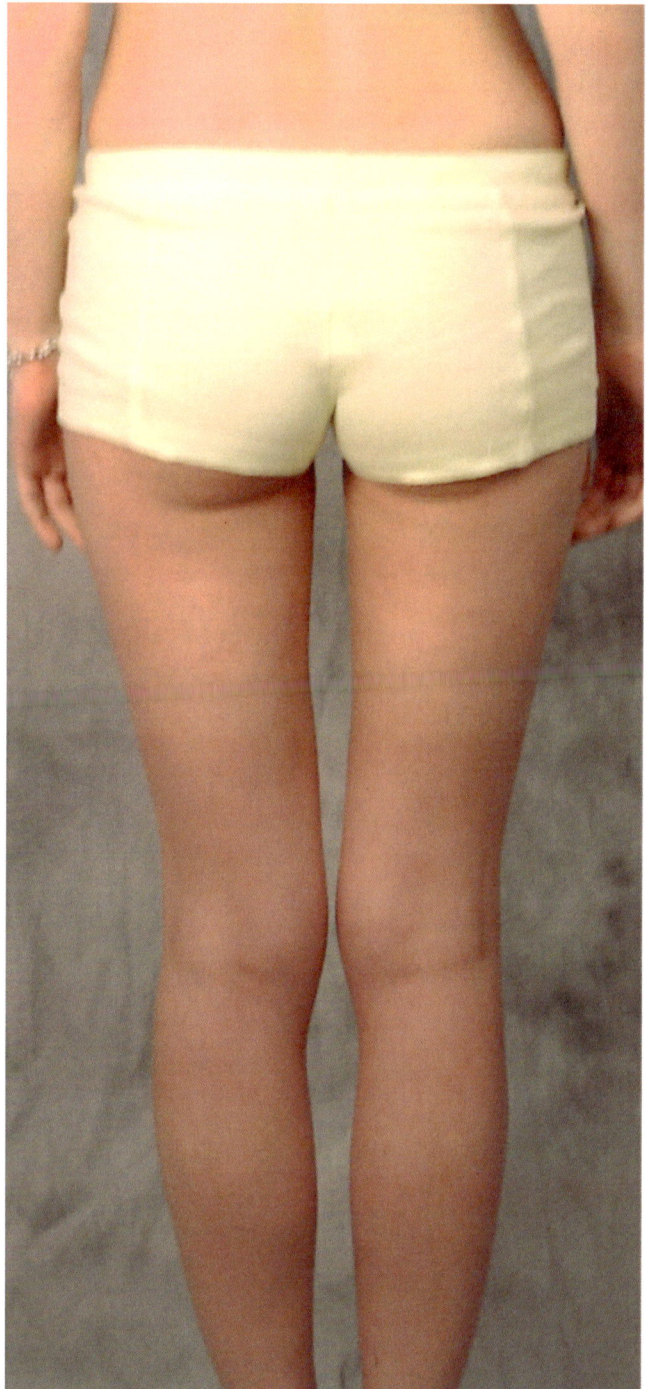

Figure P41A is a photo of the lower half of the lady on page 23. This lady's legs are incorrectly angled by her pelvic lesion.

Consequences of pelvic lesion in the R-R lesion pattern: Hips and right leg

A pelvic lesion affects all the joints of the spine.

Figure P42A, is a photo of a slim lady with a R-R pelvic lesion.

Take a long look at her right hip and legs for a moment. Note the areas you feel would be in need of treatment.

In general, her pelvis is locked to the right over the body's midline. This will angle the thigh at the top laterally.

Right Leg

Her right leg is angled posteriorly, which is the opposite to the left leg. This can be seen more clearly at her stretched knee.

Her lesioned pelvis is locked to the right of the mid-line.

The right overly rotated and everted iliac crest angles the right leg medially and rotates it anticlockwise. This force bears down on the top of the knee at a medial angle.

Reactive force travels up the right medially rotated anticlockwise foot. This places extra force on the lateral side on the right foot and vertically aligns the tibia. Where the tibia meets the underside of the right knee, the knee is forced medially. This destabilizes the knee.

These converging forces are passed on up to the hip joint and cause further misalignment .

This misalignment will affect the hips relationship with the Pelvis.

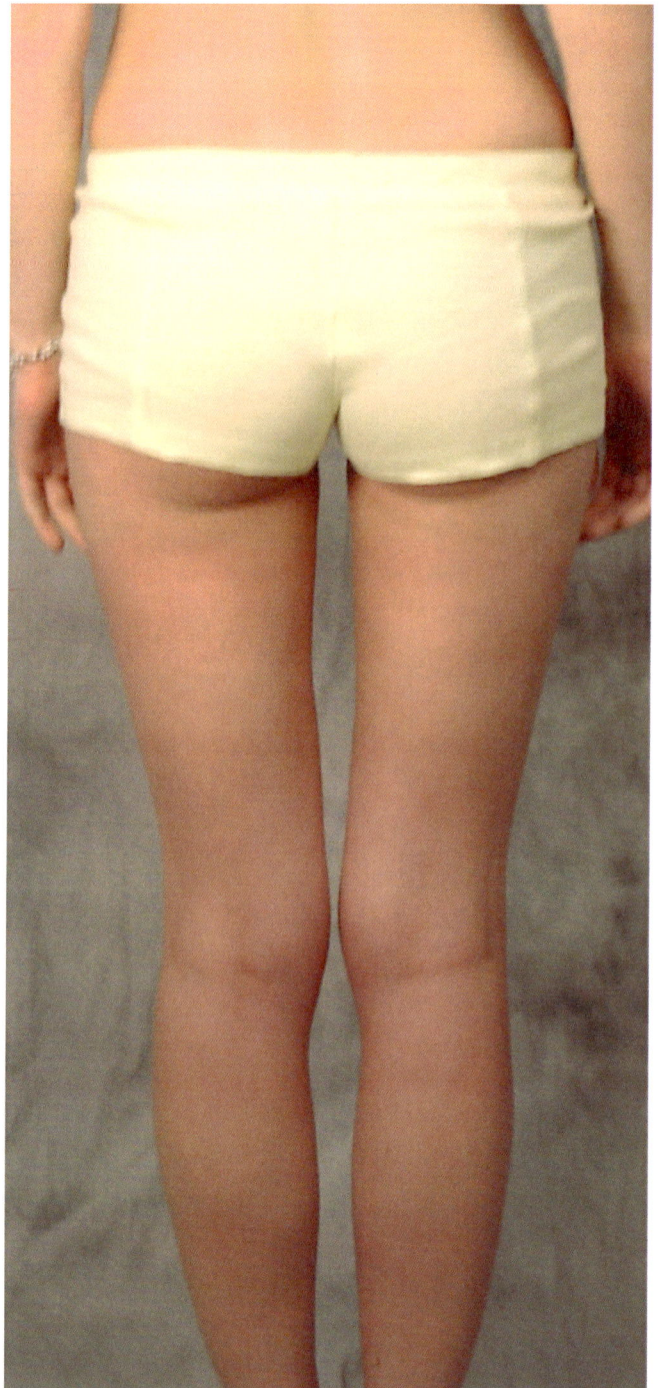

Figure P42A is a photo of the lower half of the lady on page 23. This lady's legs are incorrectly angled by her pelvic lesion.

Chapter Three
Understanding R-R pelvic lesion

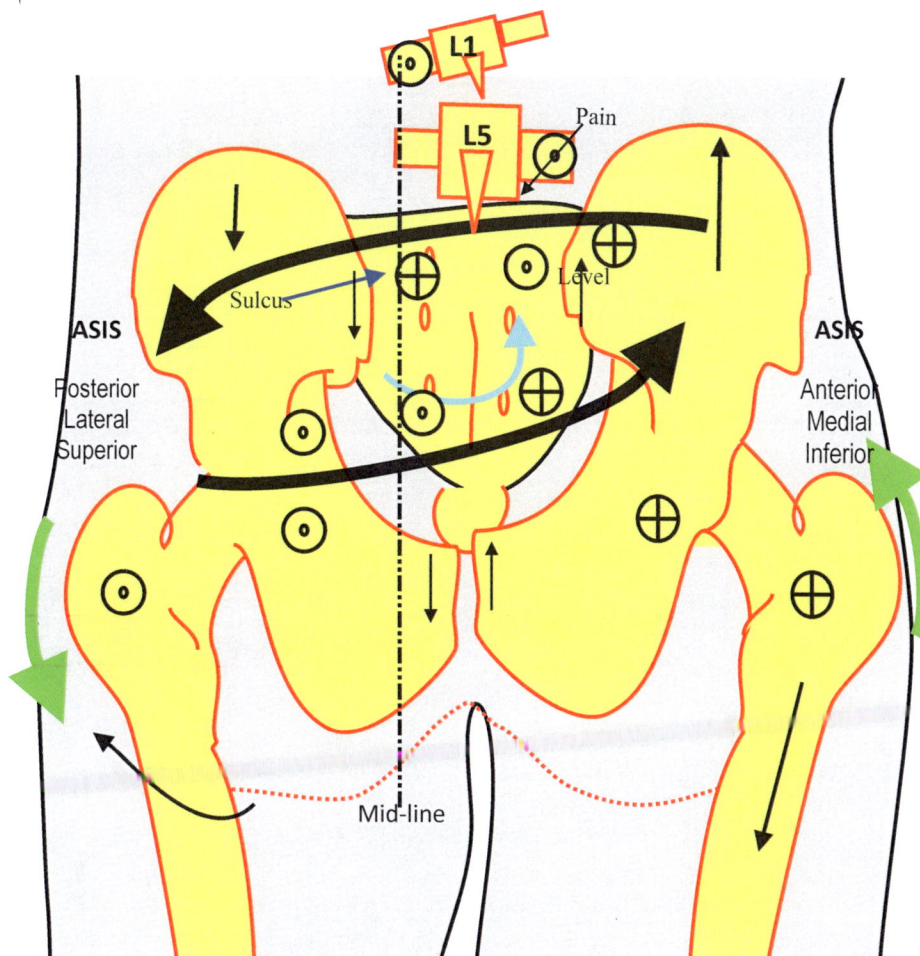

Figure P43A Key is on page 39

General

By correcting the pelvic lesion, you will change the alignment and balance of the whole skeletal system. This can put an enormous stress on all the body's muscles, ligaments, and joints. Therefore, you must know what you're doing and choose your patients wisely.

If you are still using classical techniques to correct the alignment of the lumbar and thoracic spine, your selected manipulations may not be enough to correct the skeletal alignment sufficiently to make the changes needed to make the transition. To get top results you will need to use techniques that conform to my PPT standard as set out in my book "Advanced Osteopathic Technique". PPT's get the spine to a level of alignment and mobility classical techniques have yet to aspire to, with very little to no trauma to the joint.

Straightening the human frame is a serious business and not to be taken lightly. It maybe that pelvic correction may even need to be carried out at specialist centres because of the major changes that will take place once the alignment of the pelvis has been corrected.

The two types of lesion in the pelvis

Two types of lesion.

From the pages before, it has been shown that there are two types of Osteopathic pelvic lesions at work in the R-R pelvis.

1 Facet lesions. A standard **sacroiliac** facet lesion is caused by a lumbar spine lesion, that on incorrect body movement levers the sacrum into lesion. Once the sacroiliac lesion is established, on weight bearing it will cause an **iliosacral** lesion on the opposite side. Both facet lesions can be successfully treated with careful manipulation. However, if the underlying pelvic lesion is not corrected, the facet lesions will re-establish themselves on weight bearing. See **figures P15D, P24B, P27A, P27B, P28B**.

2 A Pelvic lesion originates from the S/I facet lesions which will have misdirected the leg angles and therefore the weight distribution. On weight bearing these misdirected forces cause the pelvis to twist and lock in the S/I lesions. Pelvic lesions are reinforced every time the striding legs become weight bearing and deliver a **crab pelvis**. See **figures P28D, P32B, P32D**.

The problem arises because the bone against bone wedging self-reinforces every time a human walks, which in turn causes the pelvic lesion becomes further locked-in. It becomes a catch 22 situation. The facet lesions that caused the pelvic facet lesion in the first place become locked in. Therefore, it is no longer a simple matter of correcting the sacroiliac/iliosacral facet lesions to correct the alignment of the pelvis.

Pelvic lesion correction.

With a plethora of hand-me down classical techniques, manipulative therapists have a proven track record of getting their patients out of pain. However, the corrections were found to be short lived before the joints returned to their former lesioned position. The body is a great adapter and self-healer, so this tended to be overlooked or reluctantly accepted. Some avoided manipulating the S/I lesions altogether. Whatever, the underlying pelvic lesion was left untreated and free to continue to distort the skeletal frame and its efficiency.

It was thought that classical theories and techniques which included correcting the S/I joints together with or without articulation/massage/stretch/ and exercise were enough. And for the average patient who was in pain, it is. So, little thought was given to the overall distorted shape of the pelvis and the mayhem it causes. It was assumed that nothing more could be done .

It was explained in the last chapter why a R-R pelvic lesion goes on to put excessive misalignment on all of the body's joints. You do not have to have the brain of Albert Einstein to work out that if the pelvic misalignment is left untreated, it can lead to expensive orthopaedic surgery later in life.

At the time of writing this book medical doctors in the UK rely on muscle based Physiotherapy with blinkered precision. It is physiologically impossible to correct a pelvic or facet lesion with pills, muscle techniques, exercise, acupuncture, cranial and massage etc. By adapting the muscles to compensate for the underlying misaligned joints, the muscles will imbed the misaligned joints.

Difference between a sacroiliac lesion and an iliosacral lesion

It is important to understand the difference

I have read many books by prominent therapists who have illustrated how they correct a sacroiliac lesion using a variety of iliosacral techniques.

Sacroiliac and iliosacral lesions are not the same. Such an obvious point. So this is a recap, and is shown in block form to make it easier to understand.

Figure P45A is a typical sacroiliac lesion. The sacrum lesions on the ilium. There may be some minor movement of the ilium, but fundamentally the sacrum lesions on the ilium. This sacroiliac lesion is found in the flexion **R-R** lesion pattern on the right. It is the prime lesion.

Figure P45B is a typical sacroiliac lesion. The sacrum lesions on the ilium. There may be some minor movement of the ilium, but fundamentally the sacrum lesions on the ilium. This sacroiliac lesion is found in the extension **L-R** lesion pattern on the left. It is the prime lesion.

Figure P45C is a typical iliosacral lesion. The ilium lesions on the sacrum. There may be some minor movement of the sacrum, but fundamentally the ilium lesions on the sacrum. This iliosacral lesion is found in the extension **R-R** lesion pattern on the left.

Figure P45D is a typical iliosacral lesion. The ilium lesions on the sacrum. There may be some minor movement of the sacrum, but fundamentally the ilium lesions on the sacrum. This iliosacral lesion is found in the extension **L-R** lesion pattern on the left.

Sacroiliac lesions are the most painful as they twist and contort the spine, particularly the sacro-lumbar joints. An Iliosacral lesion will affect the nerves and angles of all the joints from the hips down.

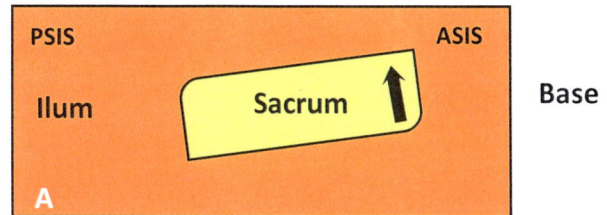

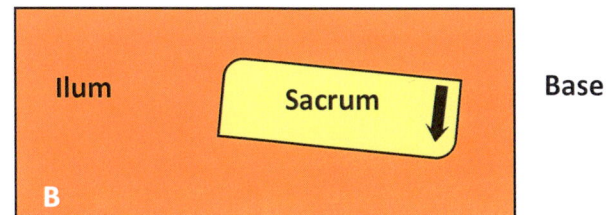

Figures P45A and B are sacroiliac lesions where the sacrum moves and lesions on the ilium.

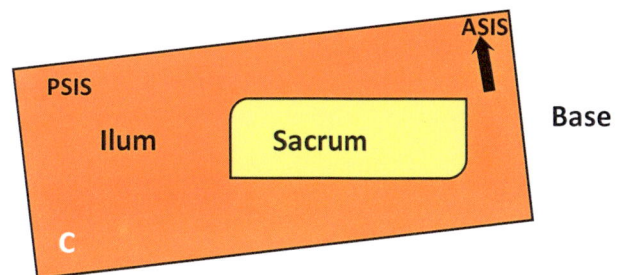

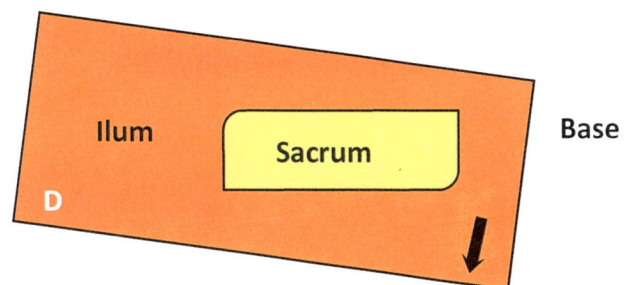

Figures P45 C and D are iliosacral lesions, where the ilium moves and lesions on the sacrum.

45

The core of the R-R pelvic Lesion.
Part one of two

The core of the RR Lesion.

Figure P46A. This iliac photo highlights the angle of the iliac 'B' and 'C' Facets.

See **figure P30A,** to remind you that the iliac facets are wedge shaped.

Figure P46A is a simple illustration showing the bulge in the iliac facets on the lower border between areas 'B' and 'C'

Figure P46B. This sacral photo highlights the angle of the underside of the sacral facets on their lower border in the area of 'B' and 'C'.

Figure P31A illustrates that in the 'F' facet lesion, the border of the right 'B' sacral facet is wedged over the right 'B' iliac facet. Reactive forces riding up the right leg on weight bearing will further impact on the Bayliss point and reinforce the 'F' facet lesion.

Figure P46C illustrates the anterior shunt placed on the displaced right 'B' facet. When reactive force travels up the laterally angled left leg, this force is transferred across the sacrum and shunts and impacts the right sacral 'C' facet to wedge against the Iliac 'B'. The Bayliss point. This buckles the joint.

Correcting the sacral facet lesions alone will not release this pelvic lesion.

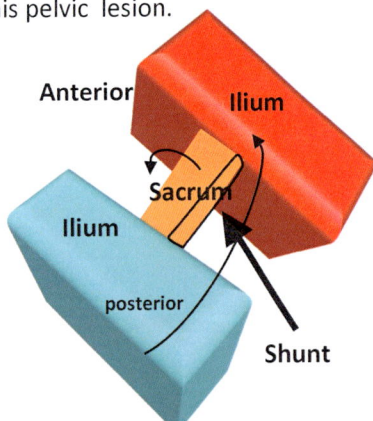

Figure P46C is a rough illustration from above, showing the torsion that takes place on the right side of sacrum when reactive force travels up the left leg and transfers to the right 'B' lesioned facet to shunt it anteriorly.

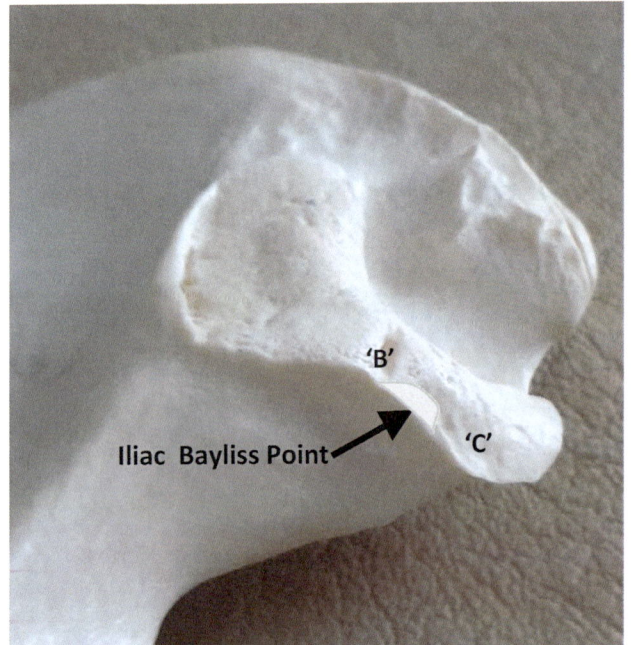

Figure P46A. Is a photo of the underside of a right iliac facet. It is shown to illustrate the bulge at the the 'B' facet. This is where the Pelvic lesion locks.

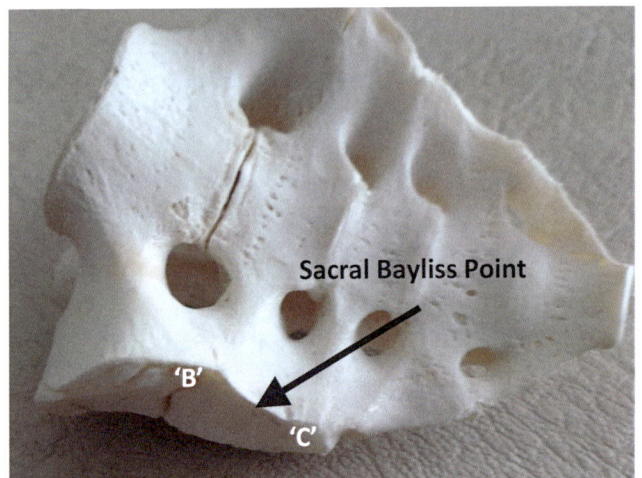

Figure P46B. Is a photo of the underside of a right sacroiliac facet. It is shown to illustrate the reciprocal concavity at the 'B' facet.

46

The heart of the R-R pelvic lesion.
Part Two of two

The right sacral facet becomes further lesioned.

As reactive body weight travels up the left leg, due to the angle of the lesioned left 'A' facet, the Prvy part of the left sacrum is force pressed against the anterior triangle of the ilium. This directs the reactive force to jar against the right sacral perimeter below points 'B' and 'C' as shown in **figures P47A** and **B.**

In summary, we have two major forces focused on the right Bayliss point. See **figure P47A.**

1 Reactive force rising up the left leg through the left side of the S/I joint bears across and down on the right S/I joint. See **figure P47A**.

2 The outwardly twisted left innominate (Left leg lateral), the body's weight is shunted forward against the Bayliss point.

With these two misdirected forces at work, with every step a human takes, the pelvic lesion is reinforced. Figure P47B highlights the forces placed on the Bayliss point. These are not symmetrical forces. The reactive force passing through the left ilium are further distorted by the left 'A' facet lesion. This force transfers through the sacrum and arrive at an oblique angle on the 'F' lesioned right facet.

Knee bending test R-R Person.

On the **right**, the S/I facets are lesioned at facet 'F' and wedged at the 'Bayliss point'. This makes the facets on the right very restricted. Therefore, when the person stands and bends their right leg, the bending movement is limited.

On the **left**, the facet is lesioned on the 'A' facet. Which is the normal facet engagement when the left leg lifts and goes forward. This enables the person to stand and bend their left knee freely. However, as the left knee bends the posterior surface of the sacrum pushes against the left bony triangle. See **figure P50A.** This in turn, it transfers force to the right, through the sacrum and shunts the right side of the sacrum against the "Bayliss" point and results in the patient feeling discomfort or pain in the right L5, S/I area.

Horizontal illustration from behind

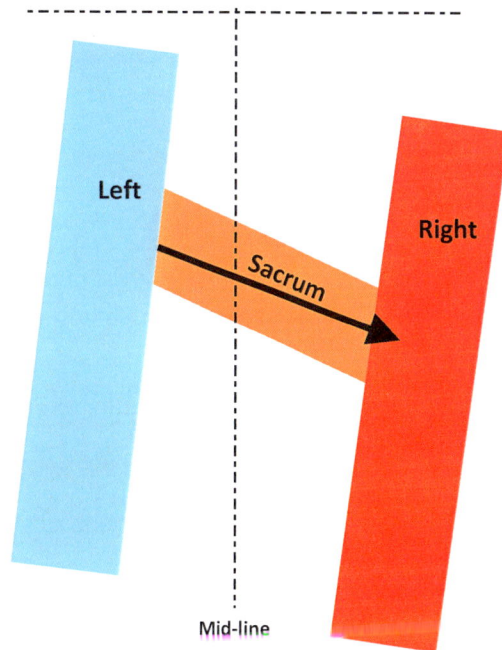

Figure P47A is a horizontal view from the back showing the angle of the sacrum as it bears down on the right iliac facets. This takes place when reactive forces travel up the left leg and pass through the sacrum to the already lesioned right facets.

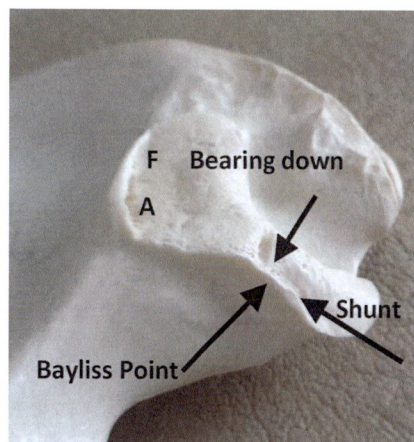

Figure P47B shows the underside of an iliac facet where combined forces act on the "Bayliss point".

Problem with correcting the R-R pelvic lesion

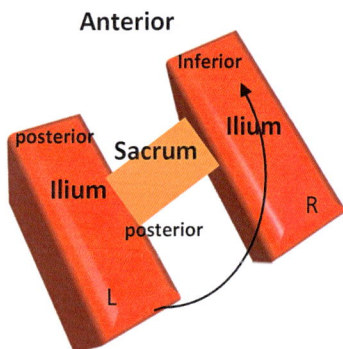

Anterior

Inferior

Ilium

posterior

Sacrum

Ilium

posterior

R

L

Figure P48A is an aerial illustration of a R-R Pelvic lesion to highlight the general rotation and distortion of the pelvis.

Catch 22 in the R-R pelvic lesion.

There are two locks on each side of the sacrum and ilium.

1) We have the already known standard sacroiliac or iliac lesions.

2) We have the bony contact where the dorsal surface of the sacrum is forced against the bony triangle of the ilium.

Figure P48A, is an overall view of a R-R pelvic lesion. In this lesion, every time we take a step, reactive force travels up the legs and the pelvic lesion is reinforced.

Figure P48B, is an illustration of the sacroiliac joint in neutral for reference purposes.

Figure P48C, is an illustration of the bony lesion at the anterior of the iliac bony triangle. (Shown for easy comparison with the other side). This bone against bone is caused by the 'F' sacroiliac lesion which is reinforced by the lateral wedging that takes place in the area of the 'C' facet.

Figure P48D, is an illustration of the bony lesion at the posterior of the iliac bony triangle. This bone against bone caused the 'A' iliosacral lesion which is reinforced by the lateral wedging, forcing the sacral 'D' facet area superior.

You cannot correct a pelvic lesion by simply correcting the sacroiliac and iliosacral lesions.

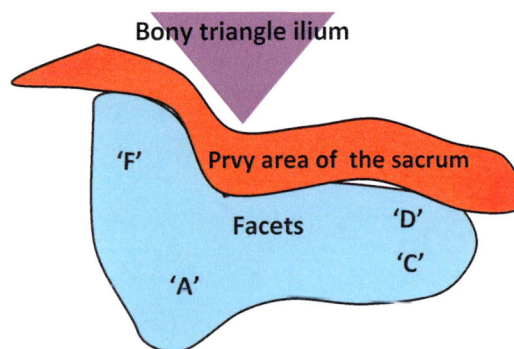

Bony triangle ilium

'F'   Prvy area of the sacrum

Facets   'D'

'C'

'A'

Figure P48B is an illustration of the dissection on the sacrum in relation to the iliac bony triangle in neutral.

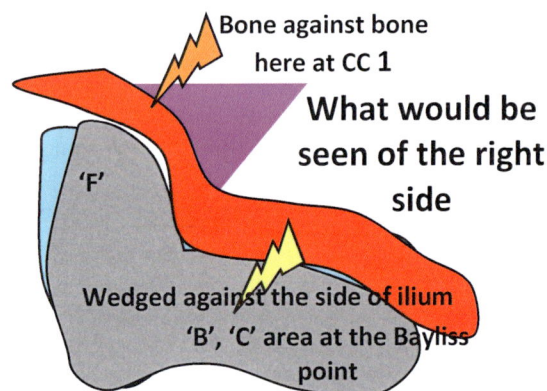

Bone against bone here at CC 1

What would be seen of the right side

'F'

Wedged against the side of ilium

'B', 'C' area at the Bayliss point

Figure P48C is an illustration of the above showing the bony contact of the sacrum against the triangle. Also where the sacral facet becomes wedged against the iliac facet in the "F" facet lesion.

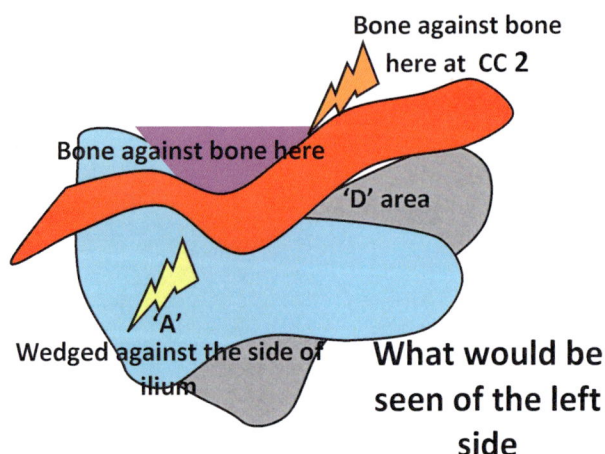

Bone against bone here at CC 2

Bone against bone here

'D' area

'A'

Wedged against the side of ilium

What would be seen of the left side

Figure P48D is an illustration of the above showing the bony contact of the sacrum against the triangle. Also where the sacral facet becomes wedged against the iliac facet in the 'A' facet lesion.

R-R pelvic Lesion - Sacroiliac facet positions

S/I facets in neutral

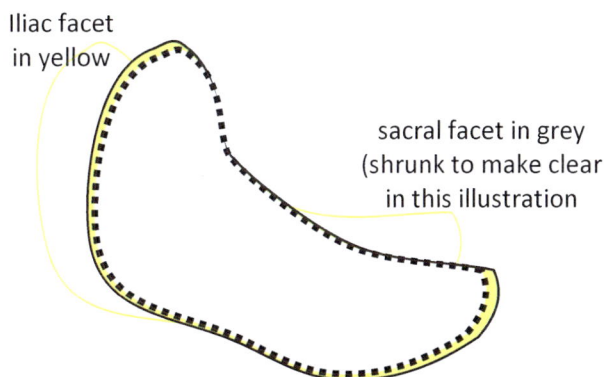

Iliac facet in yellow

sacral facet in grey (shrunk to make clear in this illustration

Figure P49A is an illustration of the sacroiliac facet seated correctly during all movements.

Positions of facets when they are in lesion.

You are referred to the valid research shown in **figure P24B**. We know that the facets semi-dislocate.

Figure P49A is an illustration of non-lesioned facets, for reference. The sacroiliac facets were not designed to semi dislocate on walking etc.

Figure P49B is an illustration of where the right sacral 'F' facet displaces against the right iliac 'F' facet, and pivots at the Bayliss point. As you can see the sacral facet is shunted away from the iliac facet. This shunt forces the sacral facet to wedge against the iliac facet at the Bayliss point. See figure **P46A and B**.

Figure P49C is an illustration of where the left sacral 'A' facet displaces against the left iliac 'A' facet, and pivots at the Bayliss point. As the sacral facet is shunted away from the Bayliss point of the iliac facet, therefore, there is no wedging.

Right S/I facets in lesion

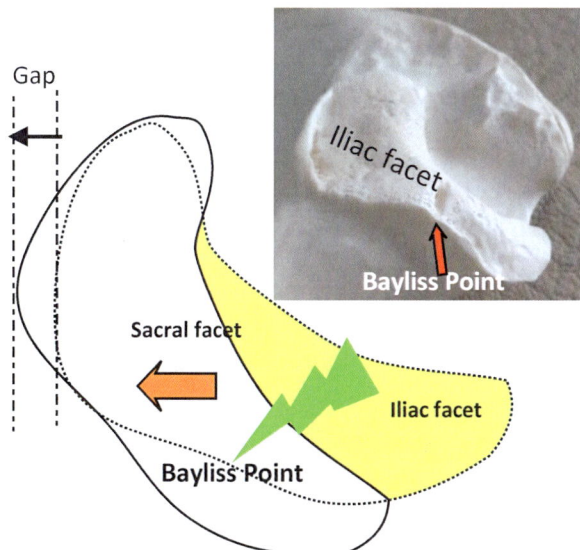

Gap

Iliac facet

Bayliss Point

Sacral facet

Iliac facet

Bayliss Point

Figure P49B is an illustration of the sacrum in lesion with the ilium. Note the sacrum is anterior to the ilium

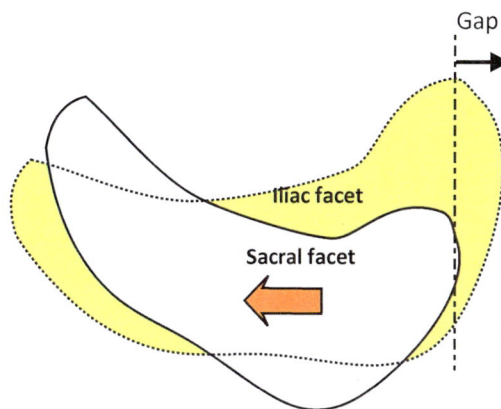

Gap

Iliac facet

Sacral facet

Figure P49C is an illustration of the ilium in lesion with the sacrum. Note the Ilium is anterior to the sacrum.

Problem associated with correcting a sacroiliac lesion on the right.

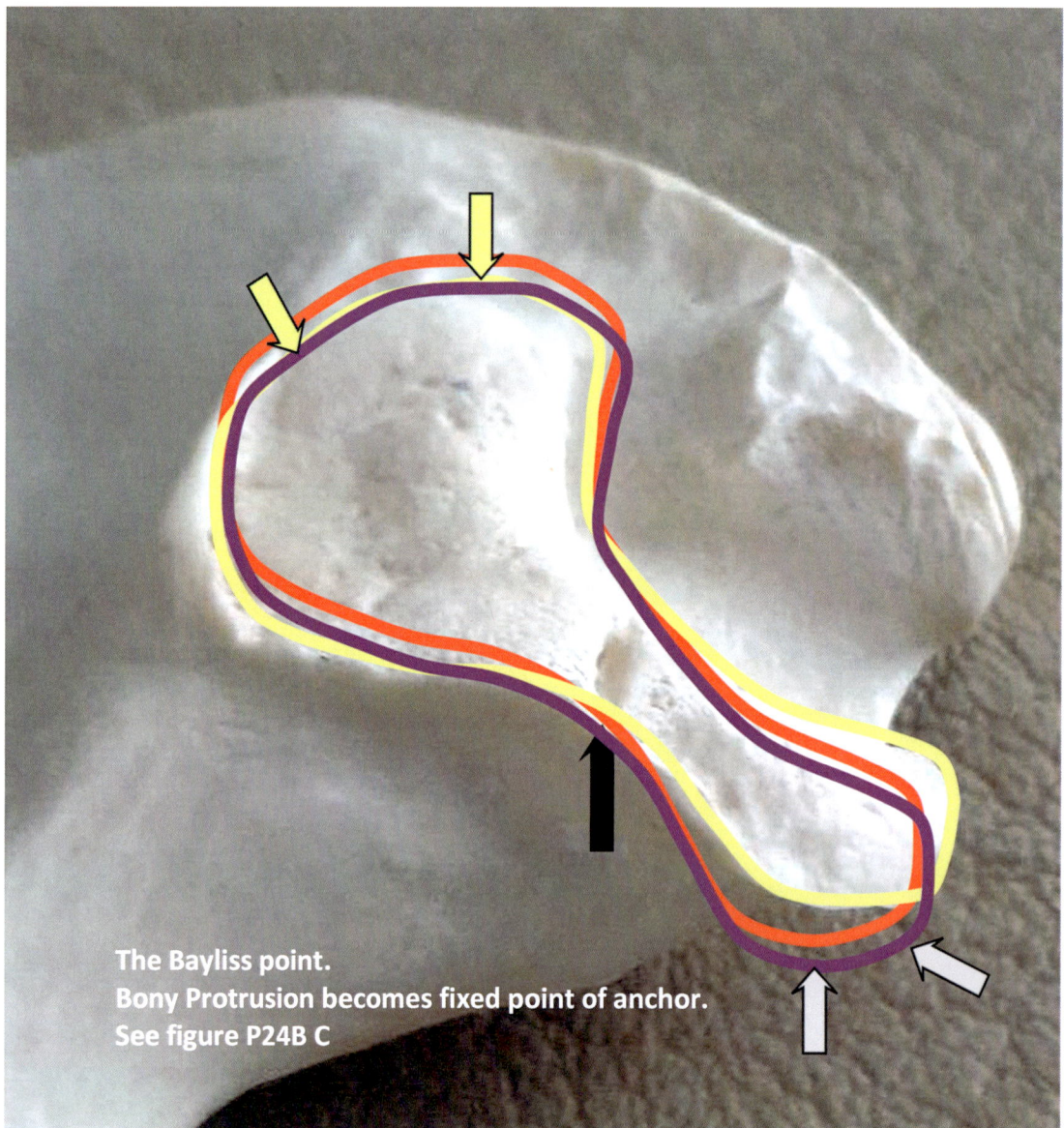

The Bayliss point.
Bony Protrusion becomes fixed point of anchor.
See figure P24B C

Figure P50A is a crude illustration of the right sacroiliac lesion in various stages. The yellow outline depicts the correct position of the right sacral facet on the iliac facet. The red line is the position of a lesioned sacral facet on the iliac facet. The purple line shows the position of the right sacral facet after standard classical manipulation. Shown by direction of thrust in yellow. If the tail end of the sacrum were to be thrusted superoanterior as shown by the grey arrows, the sacral facet would wedge against the Bayliss point and the left side would be forced to return to its former position.

Once the forward and downward force is applied from the left side on the iliosacral lesion, on weight bearing the right sacrum is forced back into lesion.

How the spine and pelvis use pelvic side-shift

Figure P51A illustrates the musculo-skeletal frame positioned in the mid-line. In the mid-line the spine and pelvis are at their strongest and most resilient. Equal forces emanate from left and right and from below and above.

Figure P51B illustrates the effect on the musculo-skeleton frame when pelvic side-shift moves to the left. In our example there is tightness on the left side of the spine and sacroiliac joints, and relaxation on the right. This creates strength to the joints and tissue on the left, and pliability to the joints and tissue on the right.

Figure P51C, is an illustration of a bow, (as in a bow and arrow). 'A' is the bow under normal tension. 'B' shows the bow flexed to the left. This flexion causes the top and bottom of the bow to lose height and the string to become loose. This is basic physics and applies to the musculo-skeletal frame.

Whilst caution should be exercised when treating the looser and therefore more vulnerable right side of the body, this is an asset that can be turned to huge advantage in clinical practice.

Think of the area B as a vacuum of energy.

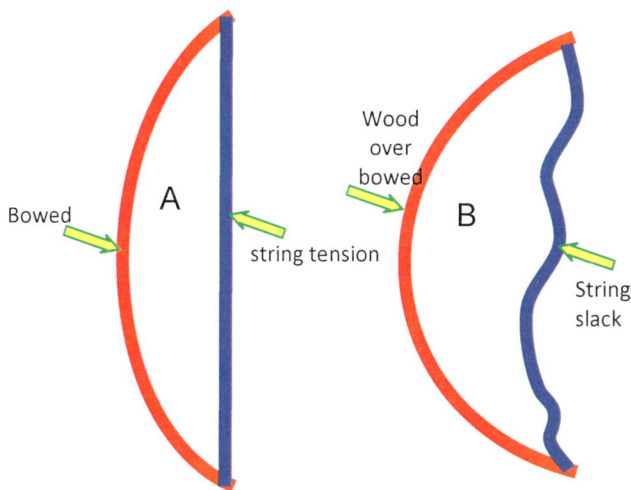

Figure P51A
This is a non weight bearing body frame with the pelvis in the mid line

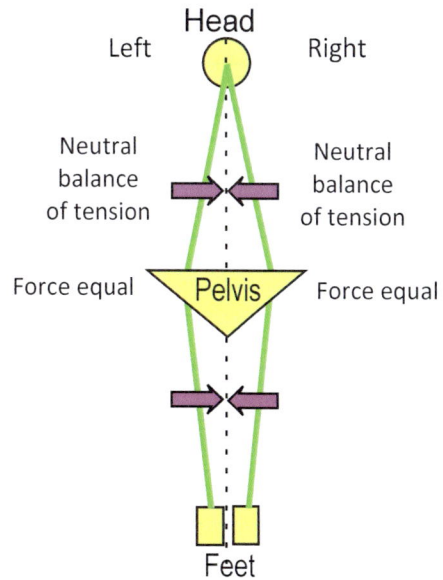

Figure P51B
This is a non weight bearing body frame with pelvic side-shift to the left

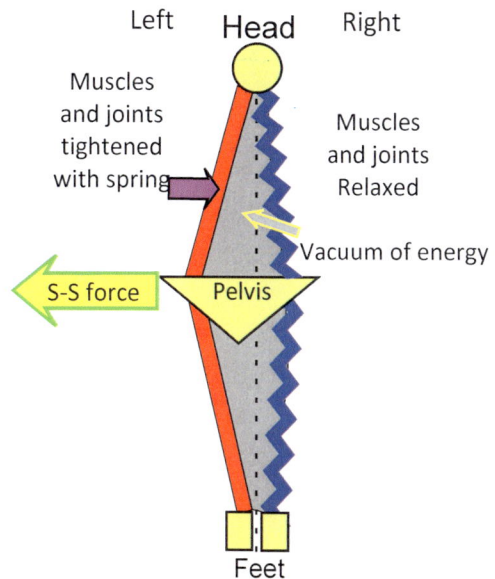

FigureP51C. The Bow Principle

51

Pelvic and vertebral side-shift

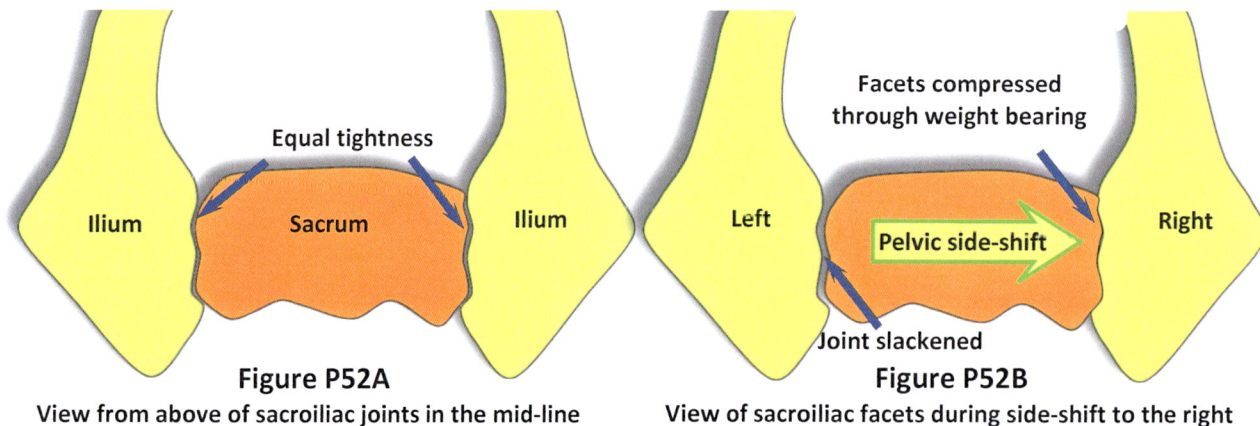

Figure P52A
View from above of sacroiliac joints in the mid-line

Figure P52B
View of sacroiliac facets during side-shift to the right

Figure P52A illustrates the sacroiliac joints from above in neutral. In this position the joints encounter an equal distribution of weight bearing and compression through both sides.

Figure P52B illustrates the sacroiliac joints when pelvic side-shift takes the weight and compression to the right. The right side of the joint becomes compressed whilst conversely, the left side of the sacroiliac joint, muscles and ligaments become slackened.

Vertebral side-shift

There is a distinct difference between side-bending and side-shift. Whilst this is a very obvious point, it has been illustrated in **figures P52C** and **P52D** as this is not a distinction that should be missed.

Another feature of side-shift is that the muscles to the opposite side to the side-shift which is to the left, as shown in **figure P52D**, become slackened. This can be useful to bear in mind when massaging or releasing tight and inflamed muscle groups.

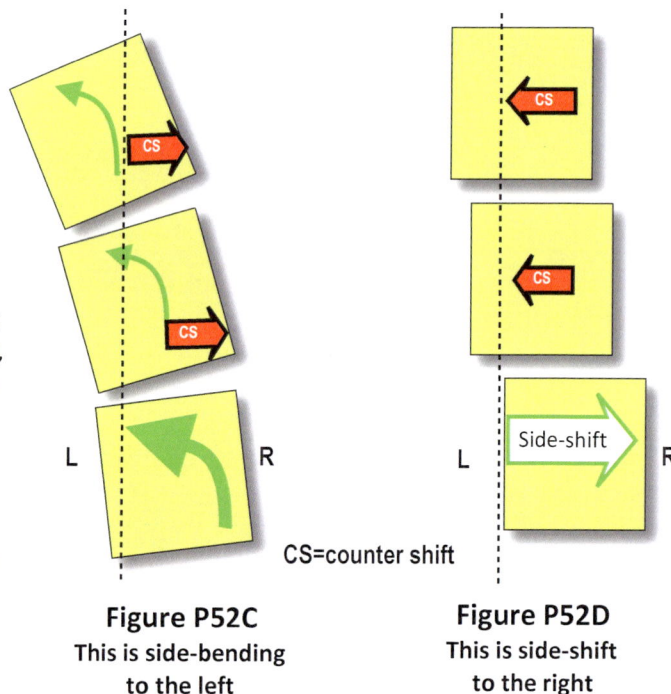

CS=counter shift

Figure P52C
This is side-bending to the left

Figure P52D
This is side-shift to the right

Correcting the R-R pelvic lesion.
The "Crab Pelvis"

General overview.

There is a rule **"first in, last out"** therefore the pelvic lesion must be addressed before the correction of the S/I joints. If this rule is not followed and the S/I joints are corrected before the pelvic lesion, they will return to their pre-manipulative position on weight bearing.

What are we correcting?

We know that the cause of the R-R pelvic lesion is initially due to the misalignment of the S/I and I/S lesions. As a result, the innominates buckle and angle the pelvis to the left. Weight returning up the misaligned left leg causes the pelvis as whole to side-shift to the right when viewed form the back. Thus, people walk around with their pelvis veering to the right, with their legs and feet angled to the left, like crabs. This puts enormous strain on all the joints of the body, particularly those that are weight bearing like the hips, knees, and ankles.

The right pelvically lesioned innominate will have angled the right acetabulum inferior and medially, to cause the right leg to rotate medially and inferiorly. Causing an arched foot.

The left pelvically lesioned innominate will have angled the left acetabulum superior and laterally, to cause the left leg to rotate laterally and superiorly. Causing a flat foot.

This set up places the left leg anterior to the right. Initially the right foot would be posterior in relation to the left on standing. However, we know that this is not what we see in practice. This is because the reactive force travelling up the laterally angled left leg twists the pelvis as a whole to the left.

The result is the right foot is levered anterior in relation to the left foot and becomes a diagnostic feature.

Every time reactive gravity works its way up the outwardly rotated left leg in the R-R pelvic lesion, the pelvic lesion is twisted and reinforced. If the sacroiliac and iliosacral lesions were corrected beforehand, the pelvic lesion will put them back to their pre-manipulative state.

To recap: The R-R lesion pattern originates from L3 rotating and side-bending to the right in lesion. This forces the right "F" sacroiliac facet into lesion. This lesion levers the left side of the sacrum along with the reactive ground force returning up the left leg into an iliosacral lesion at the "A" facet. The name of the resulting Pelvic lesion is named after the L3 lesion, which is R-R. See my book "Advanced Osteopathic Lesion" to understand in detail why and how this happens.

We have all these misaligned angles working against each other on weight bearing so the pelvic lesion becomes a self-perpetuating destructive force and becomes a catch 22 circle.

Correcting the R-R pelvic lesion.

The R-R pelvic lesion is caught up in a catch 22 circle.

The catch 22 circle has to be broken at some point if we are to correct the underlying pelvic lesion. If the lesion has been there for some time, the muscles and ligaments will have adapted to their lesioned position and need to be relaxed. I worked a way that has proven affective on a few volunteer people. It's a huge breakthrough for the manipulative professions.

Physiologists and therapists of the future armed with this ground-breaking book will now have the information they need to build on the correction of the R-R pelvic lesion.

PPT manipulations work very effectively when carried out properly. Because they reverse the Osteopathic lesion/ Chiropractic subluxation there is minimal trauma to the joints. PPT's unlike classical techniques do not forcibly lever the joint and ligaments apart or jump on the joints, which is what outdated classical techniques are designed to do. Therefore, the patient experience is far less traumatic. With PPT's there are no Kamasutra positions, so the patient is able to relax mainly in the prone position throughout the treatment session.

After correcting the pelvic lesion and L1, take the pressure of all the spinal joints which will be wrong footed. All the joints in the thoracic spine need to be corrected before the patient becomes weight bearing. With PPT's correcting all the joints in the lumbar and thoracic spine can be corrected in just a few minutes.

This amount on manipulation using classical techniques would overwhelm the back and weaken. With PPT's, this amount of manipulation is routine and in general gets patients straighter and more mobile than with classical techniques. The physics and technique behind PPT's are detailed in my book: "Advanced Osteopathic Technique".

Important.

When correcting the pelvic lesion utilizing the techniques in the following chapter, use gentle but firm pressure. The joints will move very easily. If you use the jerking action you would use in a classical technique, the joint will resist you and not correct.

As significant changes will take place as musculo-skeletal adaption takes place under weight bearing , it is wise to make a follow up treatment within 2-3 days.

Chapter Four
Correcting the R-R pelvic lesion

There are three lesions, in order of correction:

1 The iliosacral facet lesion 'A', on the left.

2 The sacroiliac facet lesion 'F', on the right.

3 The underlying sacroiliac lesion 'D', on the left.

We need a constant to diagnose accurately.

Checking the leg lengths has minimal diagnostic accuracy and cannot be relied on as there are too many variables that could cause the leg differences.

Figure P55A is a photo of the fingers in the diagnostic position.

All initial diagnosis it carried out in the mid-line.

Figure P55B. The sides of the fingers are placed under the patient's ASIS's. The pelvis is then levelled so the ASIS's are the same distance from the couch. It does not matter if the ASIS's are superior or inferior, as we just need one diagnostic measurement that can be relied on.

With the ASIS's aligned in the anterio-posterior plane, all the pelvically lesioned joints and anomalies will be highlighted on the posterior of the pelvis, and can therefore be easily palpated with some accuracy.

Figure P55C A shows how patients tend to get on the couch. Such a position if left unchecked will confuse palpatory results.

Figure P55C B shows the patient square to the couch with a cushion under their feet, so that their leg and ankle muscles can relax. This is the position you need your patient to be in for your diagnosis and treatment.

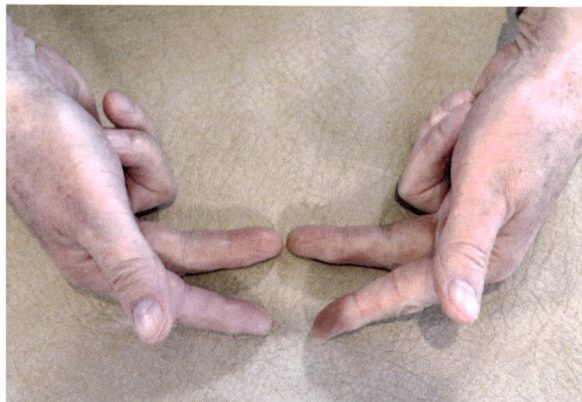

Figure P55A The fingers make an accurate diagnostic tool.

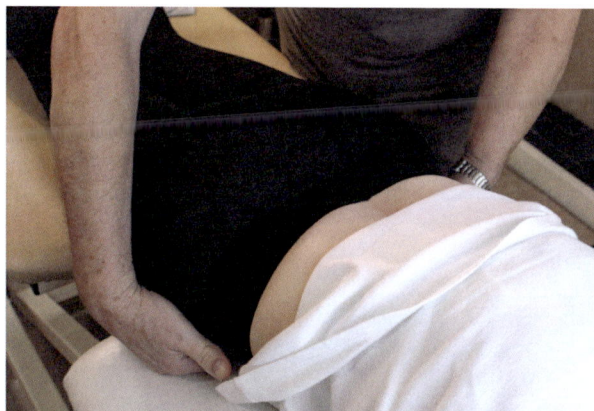

Figure P55B The fingers are placed under the ASIS's on both sides to be aligned.

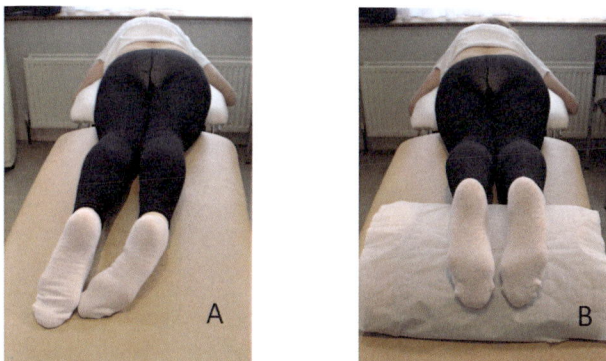

A

B

Figure P55C A and B.

Diagnosis

Accurate diagnosis is essential.

Figure P56A illustrates how to test the pelvic position. Place the palms of both hands on the patient's hips and feel which way they move the easiest. In the RR the direction of the pelvic lesion is shown in blue, and the momentum will be as shown orange. (If it was a L-R pelvic lesion, the direction of the pelvis and momentum are shown in dotted grey).

Figure P56B illustrates how to test the momentum of the legs in the R-R legs in orange. The left leg momentum will be inferior. The right leg superior. The momentum of the L-R legs is shown in dotted grey.

Figure P56C illustrates how to test the momentum of L1. Place your palm over L1 lightly and feel which way the joint is side-bending. The local tissue will tell you.

In the R-R pelvic lesion L1 will side-bend to the left. (In the L-R pelvis the side-bending will be to the right).

Figure P56D illustrates the position of the sulci in the R-R pelvic lesion. The left side will be deep, and the right almost level. The left sacral apex will be

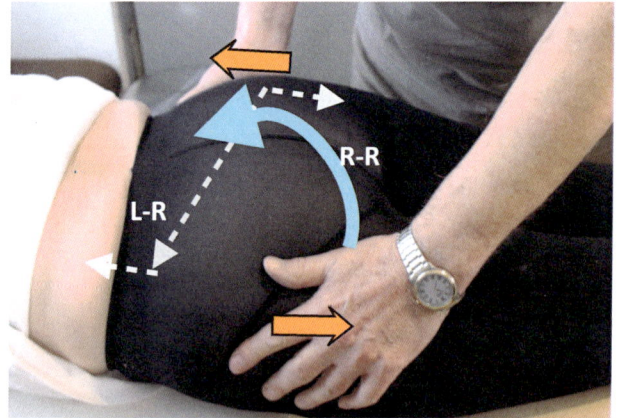

Figure P56A shows the diagnosis of the direction of the R-R pelvic lesion. Shown in blue. The dotted grey line is the direction of the L-R pelvic lesion.

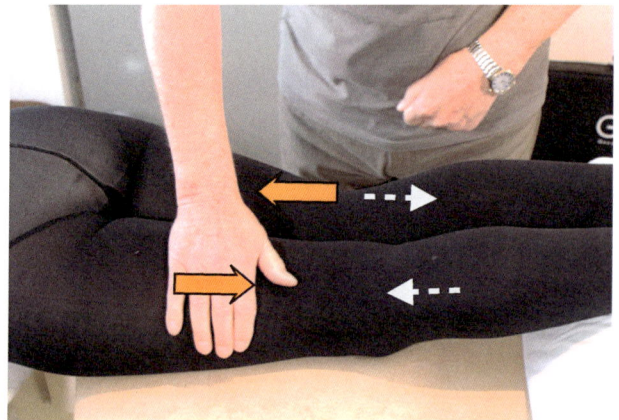

Figure P56B shows the diagnosis of the momentum the pelvic lesion creates on the legs.

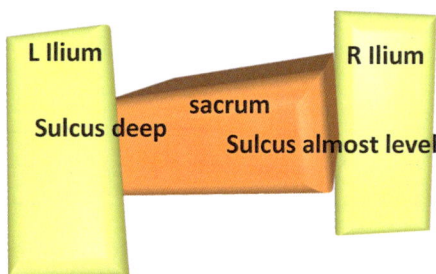

Figure P56D illustrates the position on the sacroiliac sulci with the patient prone.

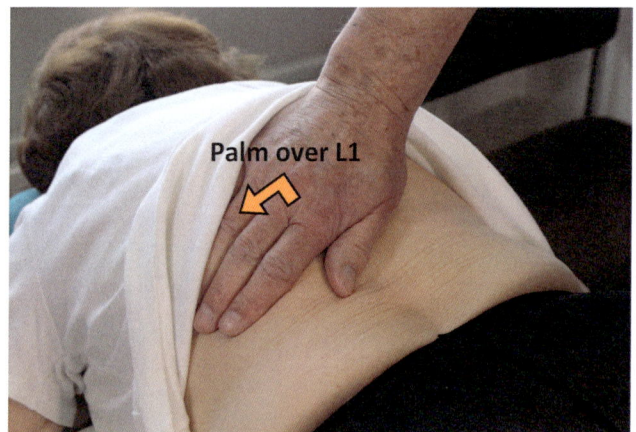

Figure P56C shows the diagnosis of the angle of L1. Side-bending will be to the left.

Placing the patient in the correct position for pelvic manipulation

Last one in, first one out.

Figure P57A. We are going to start by correcting the left iliosacral lesion.

In the R-R pelvic lesion, the pelvis will have side-shifted to the right. Therefore, we side-shift the pelvis to the right. This causes the left side of the pelvis to be on the concavity, which will be the weaker side where the muscles and ligaments are at their weakest.

(If we were correcting a L-R pelvis, the pelvis would be side-shifted to the left, on the side of the sacroiliac lesion).

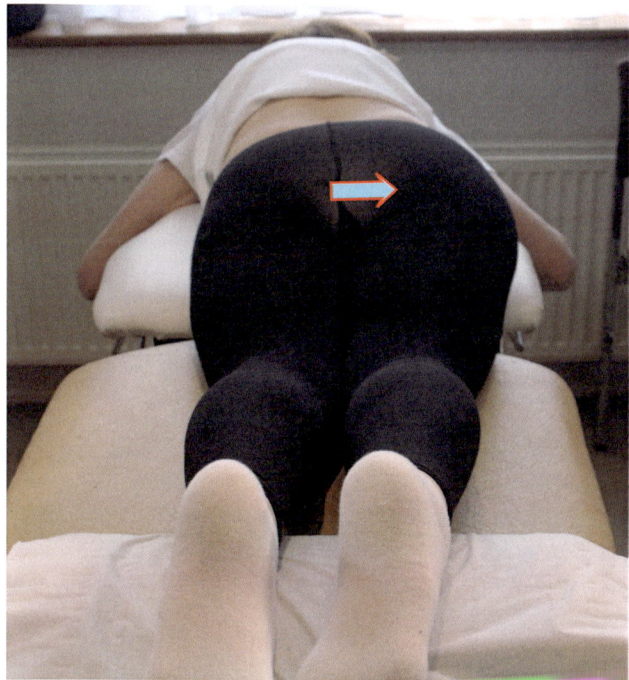

Figure P57A, shows the patient's pelvic side-shift position the patient is placed in to begin correcting the RR pelvic lesion.

Figure P57B, shows a wedge placed under the patient's left hip. This wedge offers a firm point of pivot for the manipulation over the "A" facet that is to follow.

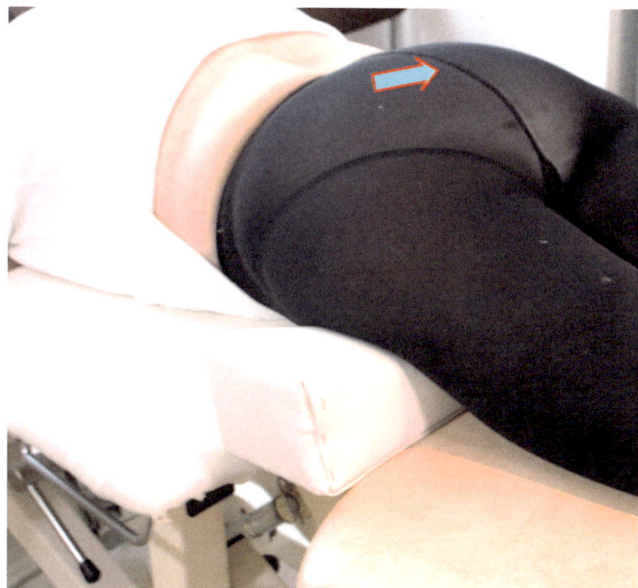

Figure P57B, shows a wedge placed under the left hip joint.

Iliosacral manipulative correction.

Manipulating the left Iliosacral lesion.

1 The iliosacral lesion on the left

Figure P58A, shows the therapist checking the momentum of the left thigh. At this point the momentum will be inferior in the R-R.

Gently pull the left leg inferiorly until the momentum is neither inferior nor superior. This will be the point of balance where the joint is correctly aligned. This is essential.

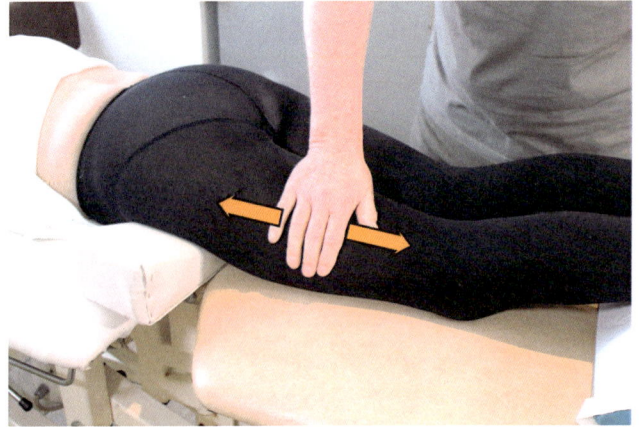

Figure P58A shows the therapist checking the momentum of the left thigh.

Figure P58B, shows the iliosacral manipulation taking place. The patient is asked to lift their upper half of torso off the couch.

The therapist gently pushes down on the left PSIS in a flowing   laterosuperior roll. Be gentle and firm, and the joint will correct very easily. If you thrust, you will lock the   joint and fail. (Remember PPT's undo the lesion, not force it apart).

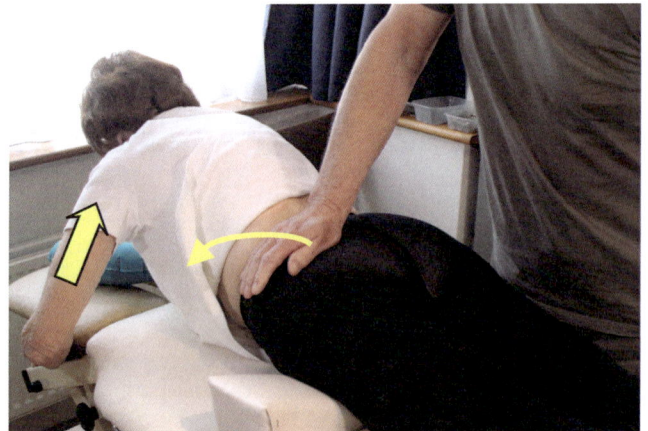

Figure P58B shows the shows the iliosacral manipulation taking place.

Sacroiliac pelvic manipulative correction. Preparation.

Manipulating the sacroiliac lesion

Figure P59A. To correctly align the right sacroiliac joint, the distal end of the couch should be lowered.

Ideally, the left leg would have a cushion under the knee to raise the left leg to compliment the alignment of the right S/I joint as shown in the small photo within figure P59A.

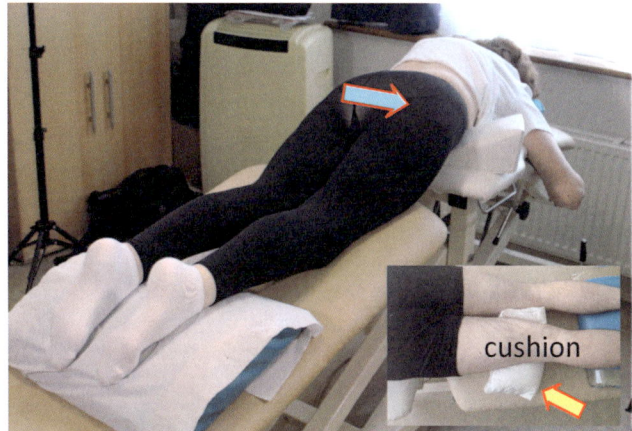

cushion

Figure P59A shows the distal end of the couch lowered in preparation for the S/I adjustment.

Figure P59B, shows the wedge placed under the right ASIS in preparation for the sacroiliac adjustment to follow.

It is important to check the right leg momentum to find the balanced position. This usually means, the right leg will need to be eased superiorly.

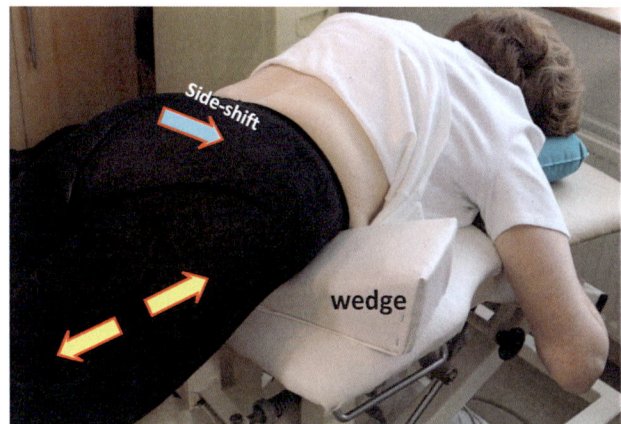

Side-shift

wedge

Figure P59B shows the distal end of the couch lowered in preparation for the S/I adjustment.

Sacroiliac pelvic lesion manipulative correction. The sacral apex.

Manipulating the right sacroiliac lesion.

Figure P60A, illustrates where the therapist's fingertips slip under the right sacral apex. It is important that you get a good purchase underneath as you will be lifting this area.

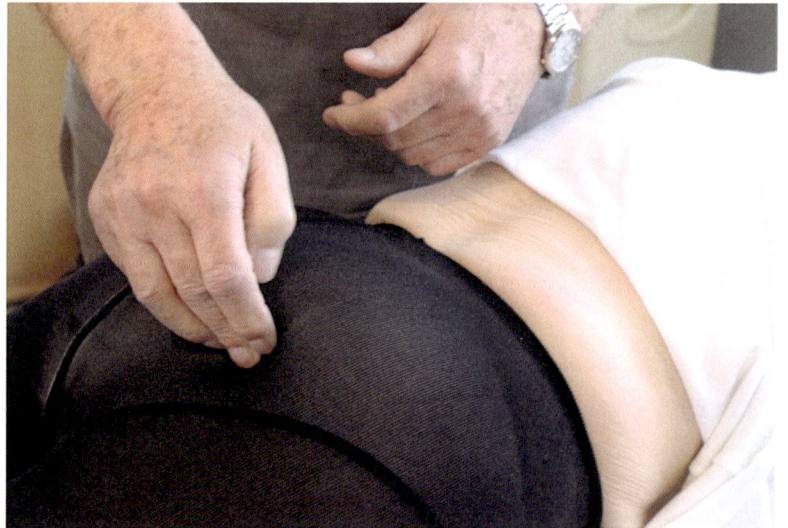

Figure P60A illustrates where the tips of your fingers go under the apex of the right sacrum.

Figure P60B, Illustrates on a plastic sacrum the point of purchase on the right side. This is approximately an inch and a half, (3.5 cm) above the patient's anus. If you are not familiar with this point, slide your fingertips down from the right sulcus. You come across it quicker than you think.

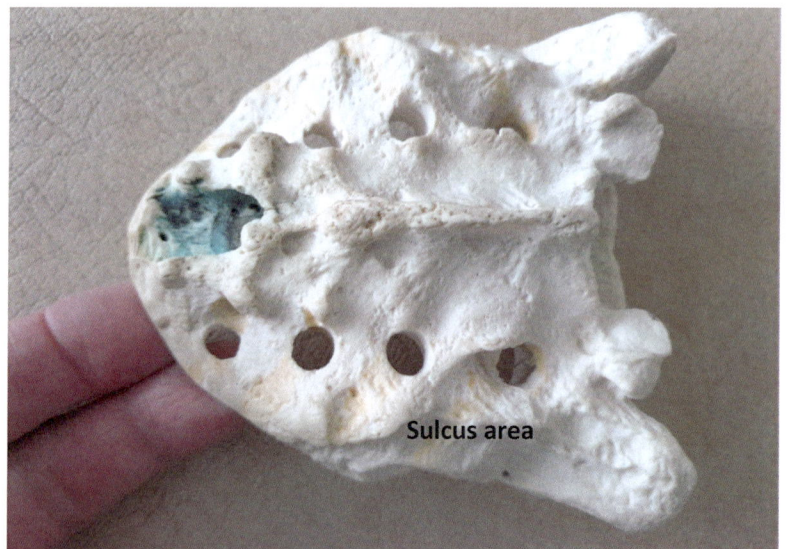

Sulcus area

Figure P60B illustrates where the tips of your fingers go under the apex of the right sacrum.

Sacroiliac pelvic lesion manipulative correction.

Manipulating the sacroiliac joint on the right.

2 **The sacroiliac lesion on the right.**

Figure P61A shows the position of the manipulating hands on the sacrum. Your action must be a flowing movement, with no jerking or thrusting.

There is an order to this movement numbered on the photo. In a nutshell:

1 Lift the apex of the sacrum over the Bayliss point.

2 Ease the sacrum inferiorly on the right.

3 Press down on the base of the sacrum to correct the alignment of the sacroiliac facet.

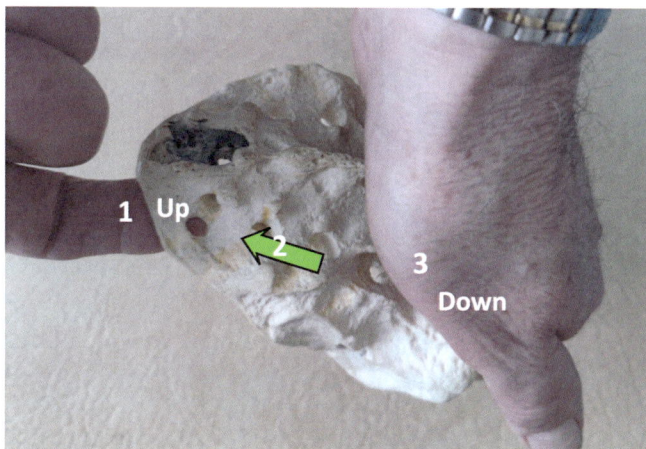

Figure 61A illustrates where the tips of your fingers slip under the apex of the sacrum.

Figure P61B is a photo of the sacroiliac joint about to be actually manipulated. See **figure P59B**.

In this demonstration the therapist stands on the left of the sacrum (It does not matter what side you stand, or which of your hands you use. The principle is the same).

The left hand is placed on the base of sacrum and holds the right base to press the ilium against the wedge. This provides a fixed point of lever, where the finger tips of the right hand can lift the apex of the sacrum.

1 The sacral apex is pried superiorly off the Bayliss point.

2 The left and right hands ease the right side of the sacrum inferiorly to further free the Bayliss point.

3 Press the base of the sacrum anteriorly with the right hand to correct the facet lesion.

It is important to make your three point manipulation firm with no sudden jerks, and in one flowing motion.

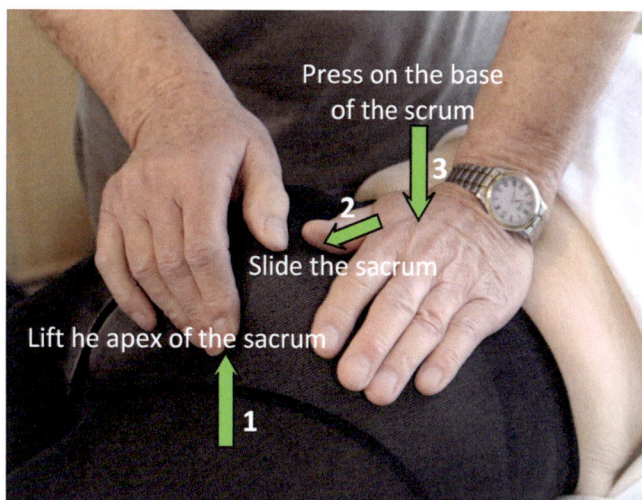

Figure 61B illustrates the hand positions. One hand on the apex of the sacrum and one on the base of the sacrum.

Iliosacral pelvic lesion manipulative correction.

Return to the left side.

3 the underlying sacroiliac lesion on the left.

We now go back to treating the iliosacral lesion where the apex of the sacrum will still be posterior.

Figure P62A shows the patient has side-shifted her pelvis to the left, and a wedge is placed under the left hip. See **figure P62B**.

Figure P62B. Shows how the posterior sacral apex on the left manipulation is manipulated. **Warning!** Do not attempt to do this technique without going through the aforementioned procedure.

In the photo the therapist is standing on the left of the patient:

The patient lifts their upper torso to lever the 'A' facet posteriorly towards the 'F' facet.

Correct the momentum of <u>both</u> legs.

Place the left hand hyperthenar eminence over the left PSIS and press down to stabilize.

Place the heel of the right hand over the left apex of the sacrum over the sacroiliac 'D' facet lesion, see **figure P65C**, and ease down in the direction of the sacral apex.

Next, correct <u>all</u> the joints in the spine and then ask the patient to stand and take a couple of steps both forwards and backwards. This puts gravity on the spine and highlights any deeper seated abnormalities.

Check the alignment of the pelvis and legs. Depending on the result you may need to repeat the procedure.

The beauty of PPT's is that they cause minimal trauma to the joints, as they unwind the joint and do not force or jar it apart. This makes it safe to repeat.

Caution. This is not a procedure to be rushed. Take great care and you will get very impressive results every time.

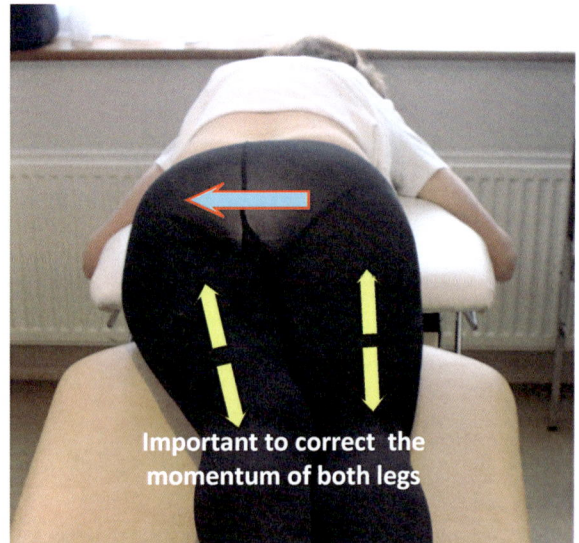

Important to correct the momentum of both legs

Figure 62A The pelvis is side shifted to the left.

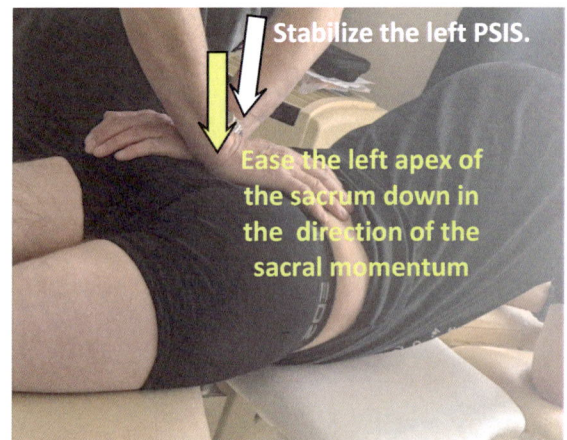

Stabilize the left PSIS.

Ease the left apex of the sacrum down in the direction of the sacral momentum

Figure 62B The heal of the therapists hand is placed over the left PSIS to stabilize the ilium. The therapists other hand is placed over the left sacral apex and eased down in the direction of the sacral momentum.

Skeleton
L3-Right-Right Subluxation Pattern

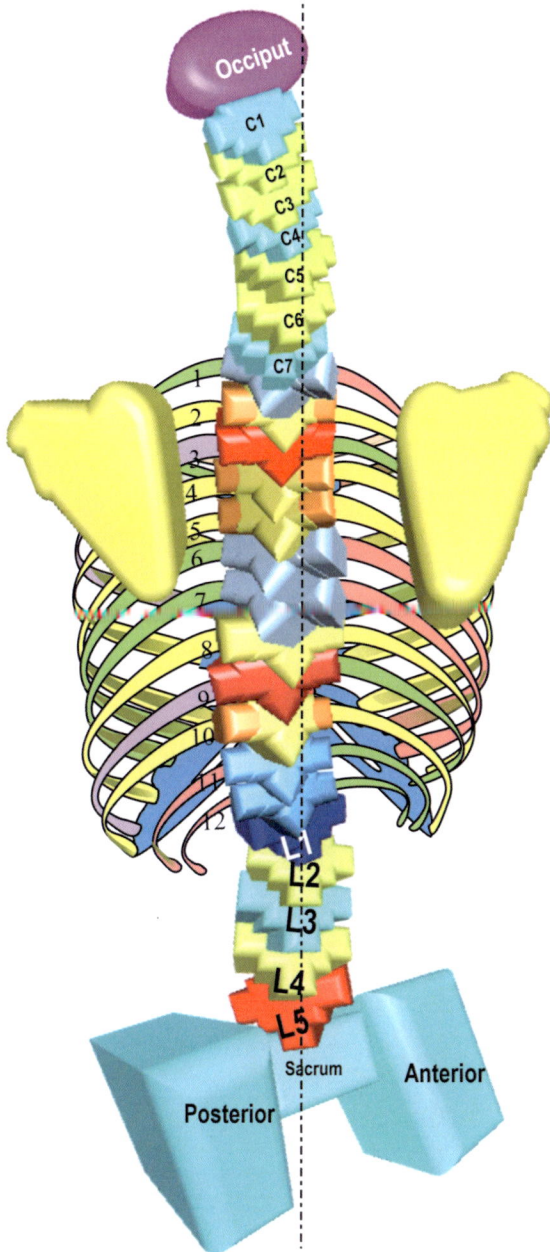

Figure P63A shows a typical R-R block diagram of the spine and pelvis .

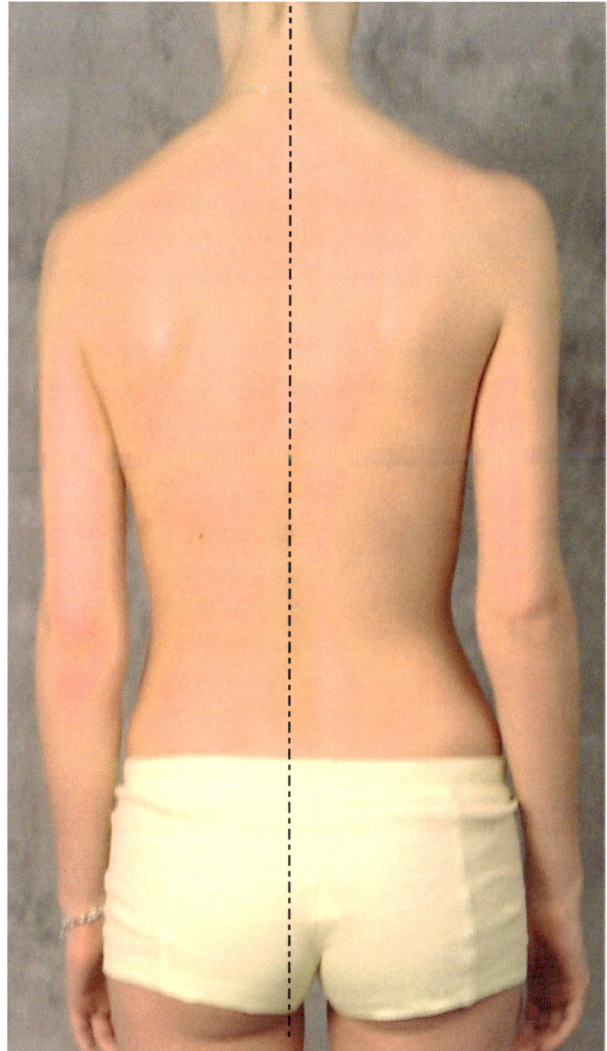

Figure P64B shows a typical R-R back

Skeleton
L3-Left-Right lesion pattern

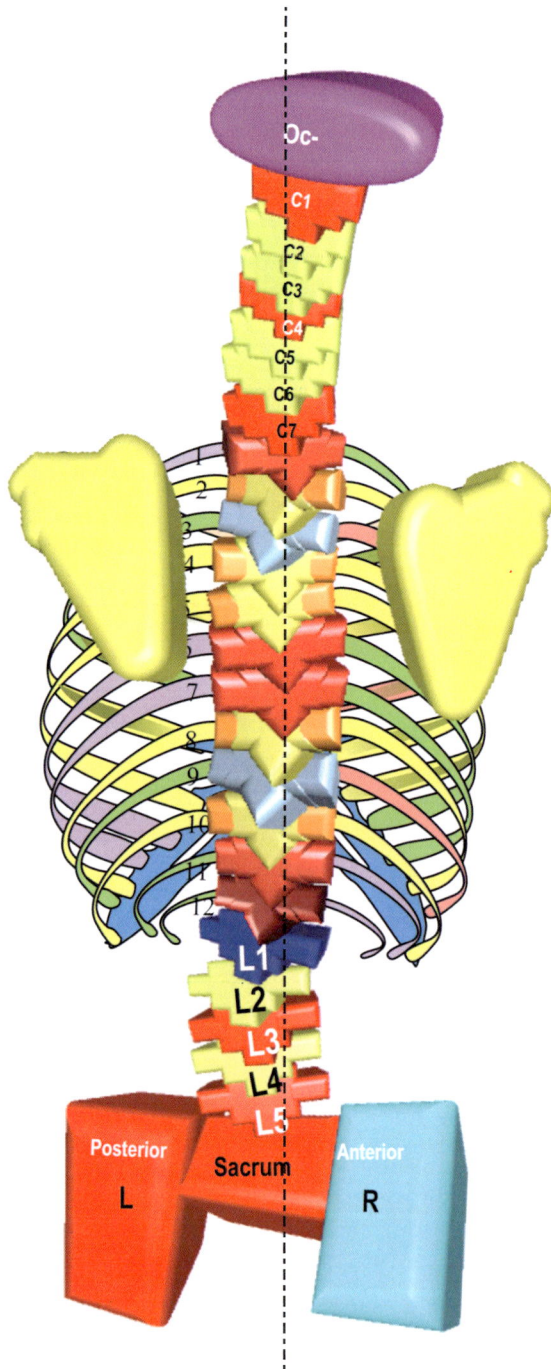

Figure P64A shows a typical L-R block diagram of the spine and pelvis

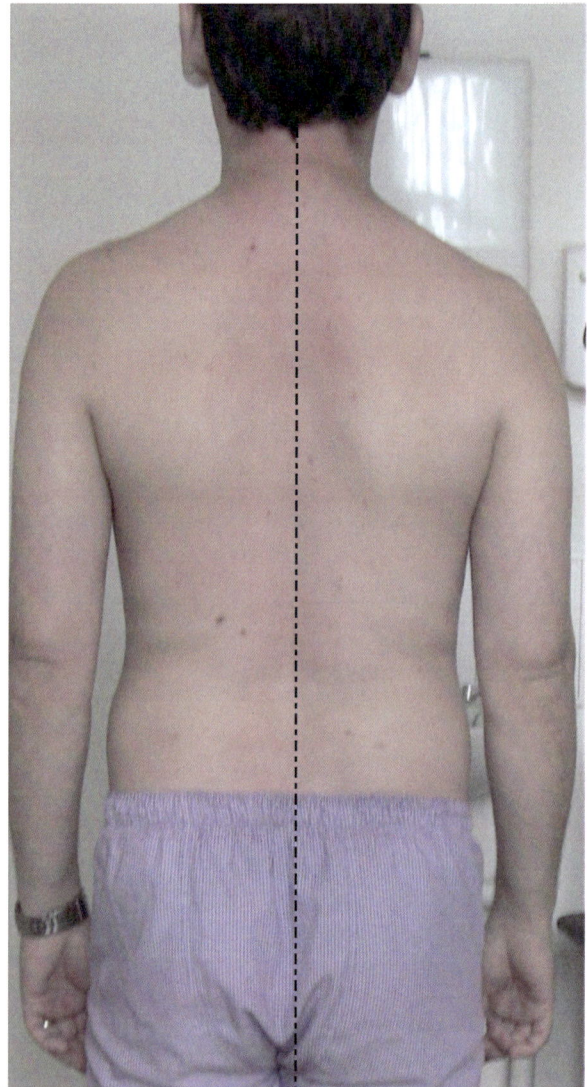

Figure P64B shows a typical L-R back

Recap
R-R and L-R lesion patterns

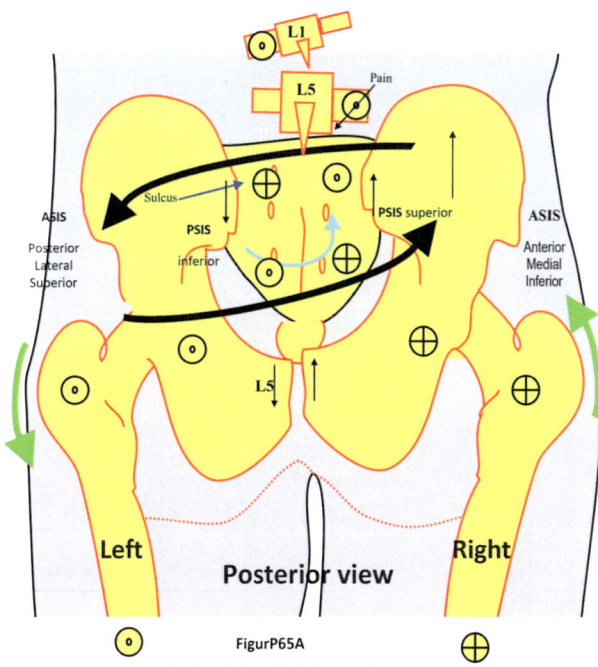

FigurP65A

Directions R-R pelvic lesioned joints
Moving towards (posterior) you —— Moving away (Anterior) from you

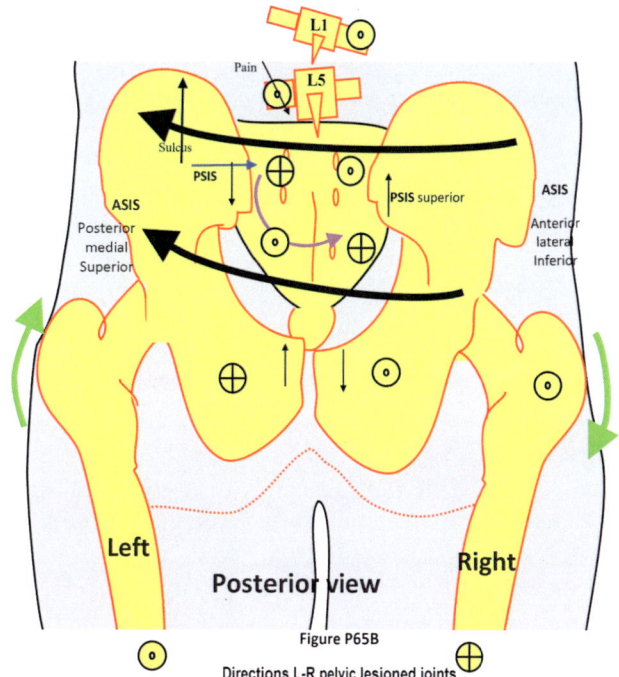

Figure P65B

Directions L-R pelvic lesioned joints
Moving towards (posterior) you —— Moving away (Anterior) from you

R-R

Side view of Sacroiliac facets

L-R

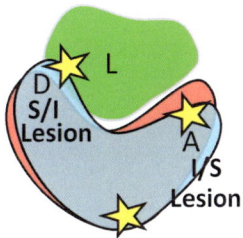

Figure P65C
lesioned left
I/S facets

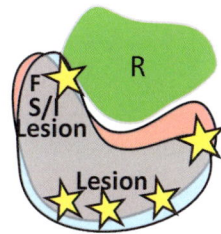

Figure P65D
lesioned right S/I
facets

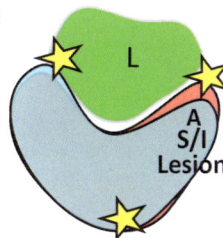

Figure 65E
lesioned left S/I
facets

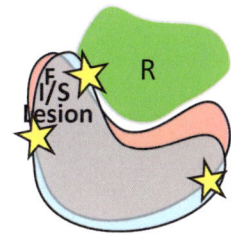

Figure P65F
lesioned right I/S
facets

Arch increased

Arch flattened

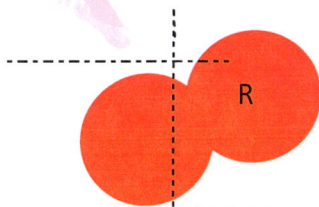

When standing

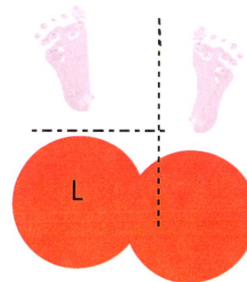

Figure P65G RR
Feet positions

Figure P65H LR
Feet positions

65

Glossary

Momentum: Imagine a car parked on a hill facing downhill. If you push the car up the hill from the front. You feel only resistance. If you push the back of the car downhill, there would be a feeling of give. The momentum is downhill. Ligaments are designed to bind joints by pulling them together and are subject to momentum forces. The momentum of the ligaments will always indicate the   direction the joint needs to go to free. A correctly aligned joint has equal momentum. Equal momentum is the position you want the S/I facets to be in when you manipulate.

Sulcus: Is the anteroposterior gap at the side of the sacrum where it mates with the Ilium. A minimal gap at the base of the sacrum is representative of an "F" facet lesion. A deep gap is representative of an "A" facet lesion.

ASIS: Anterior superior Iliac spine.

SP: spinous process. Also, symphysis pubis when talking about the pubic bone.

Bayliss Point: This is the point/area at the lower perimeter of the iliac facet that bulges. Conversely the lower sacral facet indents to match the iliac facet. When this point/area is forcibly displaced it becomes the heart of a Pelvic lesion.

Prvy area: *Pronounced in English as "Prev"….* This is the space between the upper edge of a sacral facet and its posterior surface that can make contact with the iliac triangle.

Iliac Triangle: This is a part of the bony inner rough bony surface of the ilium under the iliac crest. At its lower border it has a bony triangle with its apex approximately above the iliac "E" facet. Its purpose is to block excessive facet movement.

Ambulation: To walk independently, without aid.

Pelvic lesion: Is the lesion that reinforces the sacroiliac and iliosacral lesions. The displaced legs create a reactive ground force that travels up the legs and reinforces the incorrect position of the lesioned pelvic joints. When the sacroiliac and iliosacral lesions are corrected by whatever manipulative method, the Pelvic lesion causes them to return to their former lesioned position.

R-R: The R-R pelvic lesion originates from L3 lesioned, rotation right, side-bending right. The sacroiliac lesion is on the right.

L-R: The L-R pelvic lesion originates from L3 lesioned, side-bending left, rotation right. The sacroiliac lesion is on the left.

Note

R-R: is by far the most common lesioning pattern seen in every day practice, followed by L-R. However you can get the reverse of these, L-L, and R-L show up in your practice.

For proper palpation, and a clean reading, it is necessary for the patient to wear comfortable underwear only.

References

Gray's Anatomy Edition 36 by Williams & Warwick published by Churchill Livingstone

Weisl H. Movements of the sacroiliac joint. *Acta anat* 1955:23:80-91

The Anatomy Coloring Book by Wynn Kapit/Lawrence M. Elson published by Churchill Livingstone

Strüresson B. Movements of the sacroiliac joint: A fresh look. In: Vleeming A, Mooney V,Snijders C, Dorman T, Stoeckart R, editor. Movement, stability and low back pain. The essential Role of the pelvis. First edition New York: Churchill Livingstone 1997:171-185

The Physiology of the Joints Volume 3 The Trunk and the Vertebral Column By I. A. Kapandji published by Churchill Livingstone

Lavignolle B, Vital JM, Senegas J, Destandau J, Toson B, Bouyx P, *et al* An approach to functional anatomy of the sacroiliac joints in vivo. Anatimica Clinica 1983:5: 169-176

Journal of Osteopathic Medicine volume 7 Number 1 Clinical Considerations of Sacroiliac Anatomy by M.C.McGrath April 2004 published by Research media Pty Ltd/ Journal of Osteopathic medicine

Mooney V. Sacroiliac Joint Dysfunction. In: Vleeming A, Mooney V, Snijders C, Dorman T, Stoeckart R, editors Movement stability and low back pain. The essential role of the pelvis. First edition New York: Churchill Livingstone; 1997:37-52

Joint Motion: Method of Measuring and Recording published by American Academy of Orthopaedic Surgeons

Principles of Osteopathic Technic By H Fryette.

Bernard TN, Cassidy JD, The SIJ syndrome. Pathophysilogy,diagnosis and management. New York:Raven Press:1991.

Osteopathy: Notes on the Technique and Practice by John Wernham published by The Maidstone Osteopathic Clinic

Yullberg T, Bloomberg S, Branth B, Johnson R. Manipulation does not alter the position of the sacroiliac joint. Roentgen stereophotogrammetric analysis: 1998:23:1124-9

Interactive Spine: Chiropractic Edition. CD ROM published by Primal

Advanced Osteopathic Technique by John Bayliss DO published by John Bayliss

Bogduk N, Manipulation does not alter the position of the sacroiliac joint. A Roentgen stereophotogrammetric analysis: The pain medicine journal club journal 1998;4 -5: 223-224

PPT Manipulation Patient Research Survey Preliminary Findings by J.R.Bayliss publication by spinalmechanics.com